Preface

This guide for the evaluation and treatment of patients with Alzheimer's disease (AD) and other dementias is directed to primary care physicians as well as to other health care providers. It is based on about 15 years' experience with more than 3000 patients with memory disorders treated in the office, the hospital, or in long-term care facilities. A considerable number of patients participated in one of more than 30 different clinical trials of potential medications for the treatment of AD, conducted by our dedicated research staff members of Clinical Pharmaceutical Trials Inc.

The guide also reflects our personal teaching experiences regarding AD in conferences, lectures and rounds with physicians, house staff and medical students, as well as counselling caregivers.

This brief book is only intended to be an overview, therefore multiple references will not be cited. However, each statement is based on a thorough knowledge of the current literature.

As further scientific advances will be made in this field, there still is the recognition: "For of the Most High cometh healing".

In the interest of fluid language we refer to the patient, without any means of discrimination throughout the text, in the male form for both genders.

Ralph Walter Richter
Brigitte Zoeller Richter
Tulsa, July 2001

D0611124

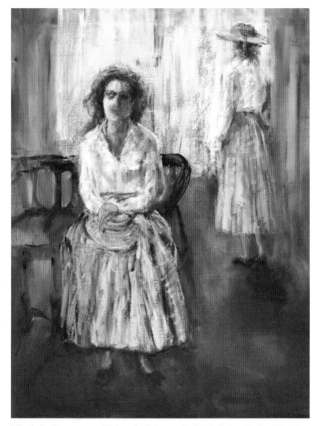

Virginia Dessauer (Tulsa,Oklahoma) Portrait in oil of a friend,
suffering from Alzheimer's disease. **Title:** *"Where am I supposed to
be now? Who am I supposed to be now?".* **Explanation given by
the artist:** *My friend often became anxious and distressed. She
would stand up and walk away. Then after looking and listening
she would return to her chair. Because of this I painted two figures.*

Contents

How the patient with Alzheimer's disease presents

Though every patient presents himself in a different way, his outward appearance, his choice of words and his expressions can offer a valuable hint as to the secret of his either bashfully hidden or (often) denied problem. There are several rather simple characteristic signs that suggest early Alzheimer's disease (AD): restlessness, insecurity, lability of affect, stains or food remnants on the clothes, a wrongly buttoned shirt.

Typically, complaints about forgetfulness and increasing unreliability are related by an upset spouse or his annoyed relative, who force the patient to consult a physician because of his malfunctioning.

Since treatment options are now available, it is of utmost importance to recognize the patient with AD as early as possible. Ten early symptoms of dementias are listed in Table 1.

Ten early symptoms of dementia, possibly indicating AD
1. Memory loss affecting professional skills or other activities.
2. Difficulty performing familiar tasks.
3. Problems with language, finding words.
4. Disorientation regarding time and place.
5. Impaired judgement.
6. Problems with abstract thinking.
7. Misplacement of (familiar) things.
8. Inexplicable changes in mood and behaviour.
9. Changes in personality.
10. Loss of initiative.
Source: US Department of Health and Human Services, Agency for Health Care Policy and Research (1966).

Table 1. Ten early symptoms of dementia, possibly indicating AD.

The patient with AD may no longer be able to function independently; the increasing cognitive impairment becomes prominent at a rather early stage of the disease, particularly in the so-called activities of daily living (ADL). The patient forgets appointments, can no longer make decisions, suffers from loss of orientation (even in a well-known neighbourhood) and can no longer handle financial affairs/budget. Formerly pleasurable activities may no longer be performed, which can result in increasing social isolation. Former workaholics lose their initiative, suddenly show lack of concern and start aimless wandering.

Abstract thinking or executive function deteriorates early in the course of disease. The patient becomes unable to solve problems, particularly by drawing logical conclusions. He experiences more and more difficulties in interpreting essential information in daily living and special situations, for example in traffic (the meaning of traffic signs becomes less clear). Typical examples of such malfunctioning are:

- Patient forgets names and birthdays of children, grandchildren, spouse.
- Patient hesitates in deciding whom of his friends to invite for dinner.
- Patient gives too high a tip at a restaurant.
- Patient forgets appointment at the hairdresser/beauty parlour or physician.
- Patient misplaces certain things (toothpaste in the refrigerator, ketchup in the bathroom, telephone in the closet) and does not remember where he put them.
- Patient does not find his way home from his daily work place.
- Patient loses ability to dress properly (wrong buttoning, undone necktie knot).

It is important to distinguish between memory impairment associated with early AD, so-called benign forgetfulness (associated with normal ageing) and a recently defined condition called mild cognitive impairment (MCI), a disorder without involvement of other functional domains.

Generally, the family or primary care physician is in a prime position to detect early AD signs, disturbances or deficits in his patients. However, in the context of screening for dementia it would be wise to consider repeatedly asking questions about short-term memory, activity level or job situation, particularly when the patient reaches the age of 65 years (though the disease can also occur in younger people). The answers can reveal certain early warning signs.

Unfortunately, most cases of AD are only diagnosed when the dementia is fully apparent. All too often, the early stage goes undetected until it has progressed to a severe and disrupting disorder. According to the recent literature, only 3.2% of mild cases and 24% of moderate to severe cases of dementia have been diagnosed, indicating that the (earlier) signs of AD are often missed in clinical practice.

Though AD normally develops gradually, there are specific situations or incidents that can trigger a more rapid onset of symptoms, for example unpleasant and upsetting family affairs, ruined holidays or head injuries.

Epidemiological findings

In former times, AD was regarded as a rare presenile disorder. At present, AD shows an increase in incidence and prevalence with increasing age. The incidence ranges in the literature from 1% to 4% of the population per year: the prevalence ranges from 3% in the younger elderly (65–74 years), 19% in persons aged 75–84, up to an estimated 47% in the aged (> 85 years). The prevalence of dementia increases with age. Beginning at the age of 65, every 5 years there is a doubling in prevalence to be expected. As women have a higher life expectancy than men, there are more women to develop AD than men in later life.

Reports in the literature vary widely about the true prevalence of AD in different countries. However, there seems to be consent among researchers about the steadily rising number of patients: the number of AD cases will probably triple over the next 30–40 years.

AD is the fourth leading cause of death in the USA. Approximately four million people in the United States currently have AD. There are an estimated 20 million with dementia worldwide (WHO, 1999). This figure gains significance when it is put in the context of increasing life expectancy and an ageing population in developing countries. Already, 66% of people with dementia live in developing countries.

The World Health Organization (WHO) recognizes that AD and other types of dementia represent a major health problem in all countries.

According to the age of the patient at disease onset, one can discern two subgroups:
• AD with early onset (< 65 years);
• AD with late onset (> 65 years).

The annual treatment costs of AD in the USA are estimated at about $100 billion. The costs increase with the severity of the disease, from approximately $18,500 per patient with mild AD per year to more than $36,000 per patient with severe AD per year. As institutionalization accounts for the biggest part of the costs, the prevention of even a small cognitive and functional decline would (due to the delay of institutionalization) save a considerable amount of money.

Causes and risk factors

The most powerful risk factors for the development of AD are age and genetic susceptibility for dementia, which also means genetic disposition for familial AD (FAD). Familial forms of early-onset AD are caused by heterozygous mutations in the genes encoding the amyloid precursor protein (APP) and the presenilins PS1 and PS2. However, the aetiology of the more prevalent forms of late-onset AD is still unknown. The neuropathological alterations of FAD are usually indistinguishable from those of sporadic AD.

The full role of the so-called susceptibility genes that influence the risk of developing AD is not yet quite clear, as genes are neither necessary nor sufficient to cause the disease by themselves. The apolipoprotein E4 (ApoE4) allele, for example, appears to be responsible for only approximately 15% of susceptibility to the disease. There might also exist other, not yet discovered genes that will make more of a contribution to AD onset than the ApoE4 allele. So, there must be other factors that are causative for the disease, such as the environment or perhaps the interaction of a number of genes.

Other risk factors include head injuries and episodes of depression. There has been much discussion about aluminium exposure and other environmental triggers, but clear scientific evidence for an association is still lacking.

Genes and mutations

The determinant mutations that cause FAD are recognized in about 200 families in the world. To date, three causative genes and their mutations in the human genome have been identified, that are likely to produce autosomal dominant FAD: presenilin 1 (PS1), presenilin 2 (PS2) and the APP molecule.

In a recent publication, a new mutation in the prion protein (PrP) gene, localized on the short arm of chromosome 20, has been described. The patient presented with a moderately progressive dementia of presenile onset and cerebral white matter changes.

Another susceptibility gene for late-onset AD, especially for patients older than 75 years of age, is the cystatin C gene (CST3). It appears to be the first described autosomal recessive risk allele in late-onset AD. It was recently identified in the Icelandic form of hereditary cerebral haemorrhage with amyloidosis. Cystatin is an endogenous proteinase inhibitor of the cathepsins B, H, L and S. In the brain, it is synthesized by neurons, astrocytes and choroid plexus cells. Its levels increase following injury, ischaemia, axotomy or surgery. Neuronal concentrations of cystatin C are reported to be increased in AD, along with its high-affinity substrate cathepsin S, which is known to cleave APP into beta-amyloid peptide.

The majority of cases with genetic background are the result of mutations of the protein PS1, found on chromosome 14q24.3. More than 80 PS1 mutations have been reported. The age at onset in most affected patients is younger than 60 years. In the cases with PS1 mutations, elevated levels of beta-amyloid can be found in the brain and blood. It is not yet clear if PS1 is a molecule in its own right, or – as it is also a transmembrane protein – if it might be identical with gamma-secretase. PS1 gene mutations directly affect the metabolism of amyloid, resulting in an increased concentration of beta-amyloid in blood and the brain. In asymptomatic carriers of the PS1 mutation, regional cerebral perfusion abnormalities are detectable on single photon emission computed tomography (SPECT) before the development of clinical symptoms of AD. Decreased SPECT perfusion can be observed in the hippocampal complex and the anterior and posterior cingulate.

Mutations of PS2, discovered on chromosome 1, are also rare. PS2 is linked with early-onset AD in a group of Volga German families, many of whom now live in the Midwestern USA or Canada.

The relatively rare gene defects in APP, located on chromosome 21, can result in dementia of very early onset (age above 40 years) (Figure 1).

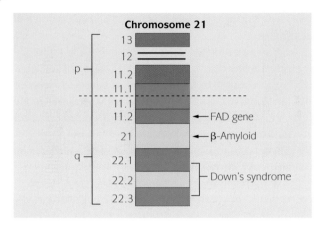

Figure 1. Chromosome 21 with gene loci for one form of familial Alzheimer's disease (FAD), amyloid precursor protein (APP), and Down's syndrome (trisomy 21).

In addition to the above-mentioned ones, there are certain "risk genes" involved in the development of AD. These are genes with multiple alleles, either protecting from or predisposing to AD of late onset. Of particular interest are the three alleles of apolipoprotein E (ApoE): ApoE2, ApoE3 and ApoE4. The majority of Caucasians (nearly 80%) are carriers of the E3 allele. Only about 15% carry E4 and 7% E2. In patients with late-onset AD, the number of E4 allele carriers appears to be over-represented. This means the risk of Caucasians developing AD in advanced age is elevated. Having two E4 alleles even means a fivefold higher risk and an earlier onset of the disease (Figure 2).

However, carrying the risky allele does not necessarily result in developing the disease. The knowledge of the mutation alone is therefore not sufficient to predict AD, and to communicate this knowledge to the particular person is a highly critical affair, that has to be handled very sensitively.

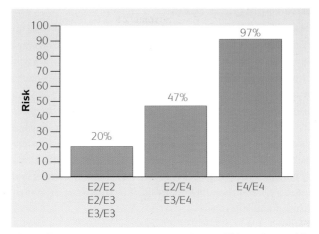

Figure 2. ApoE4 allele as a risk for AD by age 80 in patients with dementia. Figure courtesy of Athena Diagnostics.

Complex protective and disease-causal genetic factors may be involved in a variable manner for the European, Asian and Native American populations. For example, our studies in 1996 indicate that a genetic protective effect independent of the ApoE4 allele may be operative by having a high genetic degree of Cherokee Indian ancestry (who are believed to have originated from southeastern Asian people).

Mild cognitive impairment

A new risk factor for AD has emerged, called mild cognitive impairment (MCI). While the conversion rate to AD in normal age-matched controls is not higher than 1–4% (depending on age), it is elevated to 15% on average in cases of MCI. MCI is not easy to diagnose. One structural correlate of the condition, however, could be identified. Patients with MCI appear to have a measurable reduced hippocampal volume, which means smaller hippocampi, probably due to an atrophic process.

Environmental toxins

There is a long-standing discussion whether exposure to neurotoxicants can, in the long run, cause progressive declines in the function of the central nervous system beyond what is expected with normal ageing. Among putative neurotoxicants, lead is relatively well studied. Whereas lead exposure early in life is associated with cognitive and behavioural consequences in early adulthood, no convincing information existed concerning the late life neurobehavioural effects. A recent publication for the first time suggests with clear data that cognitive function, particularly functions such as learning and memory, can progressively decline due to past occupational exposure to lead.

Oxidative stress

Oxidative stress (with the formation of free radicals) can cause damage to the brain, especially when it affects the structures chronically. In the brains of AD patients, significantly increased levels of aluminium and iron have been found in the regions susceptible to degeneration. These metals may be the source of chronic oxidative stress, but the definite proof for a role in the pathogenesis is still lacking.

Medical conditions

There are several other medical conditions which are correlated with an altered mental status. Patients with cancer, for example, often have multiple causes of delirium, many of which are treatable – with usually rapid improvement in their cognitive status.

Major depression and depressive symptoms have been found to be a risk factor for AD. A relationship was also reported recently between cerebral white matter lesions (periventricular and subcortical) and subjective cognitive failures.

There is some, but overall not conclusive, evidence that moderate and severe head injuries in early adulthood may be associated with increased risk of AD and other dementias in late life. Recent prospective data suggest that the risk of AD increases with the severity of the head injury.

Down's syndrome is not yet definitely established as a risk factor for AD, but is strongly related to dementia. As many as 50% of people with Down's syndrome may develop clinical signs of AD, usually at a much younger age (over 30 years) than the healthy population. Patients with Down's syndrome have an extra copy of chromosome 21, which bears the gene for APP.

Cerebrovascular diseases may predispose to dementia. The association between AD and vascular factors may reflect some of the shared pathogenic pathways, such as ApoE4, oxidative stress, apoptosis, disturbance in the renin–angiotensin system and psychological stress. AD, on the other hand, causes or stimulates vascular diseases.

Mental ability

A series of studies revealed an association between lower mental ability in childhood and late-onset dementia, but not with dementia of early onset. This finding stresses the particular importance of environmental factors during the early years of life. Childhood mental ability may shape adult health-related behaviours, some of which could predispose to late-life cognitive decline and dementia. Higher mental ability may allow access to better health information and thus help people to make better choices regarding lifestyle or exposure to environmental factors linked to cognitive decline.

Marital status, gender and others

Singles have a significantly higher risk of dementia or AD in old age than married people. The risk is twofold higher for dementia and threefold higher for AD.

To be a female means to have a higher risk for the development of AD than a male. This controversial observation is primarily based on epidemiological prevalence data. The underlying biological explanation could be found in postmenopausal declines in (protective?) oestrogen levels.

Other established or suggested risk factors for the development of AD at a higher age include: low social and economic status, magnetic field exposure, low head circumference, lack of physical activity, severe malnutrition.

Potentially protective factors

Several variables appear to have an inverse association with the presence of dementia or symptoms of AD, which suggests a kind of protection. These variables include the ApoE2 allele, higher educational level, use of antioxidants such as vitamin E, use of oestrogen supplements in women, use of anti-inflammatory agents, use of statins and (very controversial) cigarette smoking.

Diagnostic criteria

Cognitive impairment is mostly admitted with delay by the patient and his family, and still widely underdiagnosed by health care professionals. A median of 1.6 years elapses between a caregiver's first recognition of a dementia symptom and the consultation of a physician for evaluation. The diagnosis of AD is typically made 3.5–5.5 years after symptoms develop. Less than half of AD patients are diagnosed at all. The early symptoms of this degenerative disease are often mistaken for depression or as part of the ageing process.

Early detection of AD not only facilitates an effective therapy and lessens the disease burden. Other benefits relate to the identification of reversible causes of dementia, as well as the ability of the patient and his family to make plans for the future (living situation, financial, legal aspects).

Some experts favour a routine screening for dementia in patients over age 65, particularly in women, who show a higher AD prevalence than men.

Definition of AD

AD is a disorder with a gradual onset leading to a significant impairment in cognitive function, which continues to decline over time (DSM-IV, 1994).

Once considered a disease diagnosed by exclusion of other possible forms of dementia, AD is now considered a diagnosis of inclusion, with specific defining characteristics. The diagnosis is based on a combination of thorough clinical evaluation (physical examination, neuroimaging techniques, laboratory tests) and validated neuropsychological assessment tools.

AD today is regarded as a syndrome. Among the various forms of dementia, AD and vascular dementia (VaD) are the most frequent disorders, and may often co-exist in the same patient.

Dementia disorders are characterized by the development of multiple cognitive deficits (including memory impairment) that are due to the direct physiological effects of a general medical condition, to the persisting effects of a substance, or to multiple aetiologies. The disorders share a common symptom presentation but are differentiated based on aetiology.

The essential feature of a dementia is the development of multiple cognitive deficits that include memory impairment and at least one of the following cognitive disturbances:

- Aphasia (deterioration of language function).
- Apraxia (impaired ability to execute motor activities despite intact motor abilities, sensory function and comprehension of required task).
- Agnosia (failure to recognize or identify objects).
- Disturbances in executive functioning (loss of the ability to think abstractly, to count, to plan, to initiate, to sequence).

The cognitive deficits must be sufficiently severe to cause impairment and must represent a decline from a previously higher level of functioning.

Memory impairment is required to make the diagnosis of dementia and is a prominent early symptom. Individuals with dementia become impaired in their ability to learn new things, or they forget previously learned and well-known material. The patients may lose important items (wallet, keys), forget food cooking on the stove, are ashamed of their forgetfulness of names and facts, and isolate themselves.

AD is a progressive degenerative disorder, characterized by impairments of memory (particularly the recent memory) and disturbances in at least one other cognitive domain (Table 2).

The onset of dementia of the Alzheimer's type is gradual and involves continuing cognitive decline. Because of the difficulty of obtaining direct pathological evidence of the presence of AD, the diagnosis can only be made when other aetiologies for the dementia have been ruled out.

The course of AD tends to be slowly progressive, with a loss of 3–4 points per year on the Mini Mental State Examination (MMSE) or an average yearly change on the AD Assessment Scale–cognitive subscale (ADAS-cog) of between 7 and 9 points. The disease is associated with various patterns of deficits: early impairment of recent memory, personality changes or increased irritability, sleep disturbances (day–night reversal, with so-called sun-downing phenomenon) (in the early stages), gait and motor disturbances (in the later stages).

DSM-IV diagnostic criteria for AD
Multiple cognitive deficits
Short- and long-term memory impairment
One or more of the following:
Aphasia (language disturbance)
Apraxia (impaired ability to carry out familiar tasks
Agnosia (failure to recognize familiar objects)
Disturbances in executive functioning (planning, organizing, abstract thinking)
Gradual onset, significant functional impairment and continuous decline
Decline from previously higher level of function
Exclusion of other possible causes
No evidence for delirium
Source: DSM-IV™ (1994), adapted.

Table 2. DSM-IV diagnostic criteria for AD.

Differential diagnosis of dementia

There are several clinical features that can be of help in distinguishing different forms of dementias. The differentiation is mainly based on three categories of signs and symptoms: (1) cognitive and motor disturbances, personality changes/behavioural alteration; (2) time of occurrence of symptoms; (3) mode of onset of dementia (slow or rapid, early or later).

The differential diagnosis of dementias can be facilitated by using selected criteria, already developed by a group of scientists under the auspices of the Department of Health and Human Services Task Force on Alzheimer's Disease in 1984 (National Institutes of Neurologic and Communicative Diseases and Stroke – Alzheimer's Disease and Related Disorders Association, NINCDS-ADRDA) (Table 3).

Delirium

Dementia must be distinguished from delirium, which by definition is transient and potentially reversible. Dementia and delirium are both manifestations of "brain failure". Dementia indicates evidence of anatomical brain damage, and delirium is a sign of functional impairment. The two conditions often interact.

The delirious patient tends to have fluctuating levels of awareness. Visual and auditory hallucinations may be more prominent in delirium than in dementia, but they can certainly be seen in demented patients as well. Delirious patients tend to have more tremors and other motor manifestations.

Medical illnesses and seizures frequently accompany delirium but can be seen in dementia as well. And, to make the diagnostic difficulties even more complex, patients with dementia are typically more susceptible to conditions which cause delirium (Table 4).

Generally, delirium is to be considered a medical emergency. Among elderly patients, the emergence of a delirium can also be the first warning sign that dementia is developing.

A wide spectrum of drugs may cause delirium, hostility, agitation, uncontrollable crying, confusion and severe depression. These include over-the-counter (OTC) drugs, as well as those which require prescription, and those which are typically obtained illicitly. The intake of such drugs can lead to a misdiagnosis if the physician is not careful in recording the patient's drug history, especially taken from family members. In elderly patients, higher doses of normally prescribed medications may lead to adverse reactions. In other instances, symptoms may not appear until after cessation of therapy, especially if done abruptly (e.g. benzodiazepines, analgesics, alcohol).

Delirium is classically associated with impairment of oxidative metabolism in the brain. Indeed, hypoxia is a classical cause of delirium.

Selected NINCDS-ADRDA criteria
Probable AD
Dementia
Deficits in two or more cognitive areas
Progressive worsening of memory and other cognitive functions
No disturbance of consciousness
Onset between 40 and 90 years of age
Absence of other systemic disorders
Progressive worsening of specific cognitive functions
Impaired ADL
Associated behavioural abnormalities
Possible AD
Dementia syndrome in the absence of other neurological, psychiatric or systemic disorders sufficient to cause dementia, and in the presence of variations in the onset, in the presentation, or in the clinical course
Uncertain/unlikely AD
Sudden onset
Focal neurological findings
Early seizures or gait disturbances

Table 3. Selected NINCDS-ADRDA criteria.

Older patients may have premorbid pathology, so that the symptoms may be caused either by the disease or the drug. For example, respiratory insufficiency can cause thought disorder.

Conditions causing delirium in the elderly
Infections Septicaemia Bronchopneumonia Severe urinary tract infection HIV encephalitis
Head injury Acute or chronic subdural haematoma Post-concussion syndrome

Metabolic encephalopathy
Hypoglycaemia/hyperinsulinism
Diabetic acidosis
Severe hypothyroidism
Thyroid storm
Severe B_{12} deficiency
Electrolyte imbalance
    Hyponatraemia or hypernatraemia
    Hypocalcaemia or hypercalcaemia
    Renal insufficiency

Decreased cerebral perfusion Chronic pulmonary insufficiency Chronic hypoxaemia Severe cardiac output defect
Toxic effects of medications Mind-altering and addictive substances (alcohol) Antipsychotics and antidepressants Antiparkinson drugs Cardiovascular and antihypertensive drugs Anticonvulsant drugs Anticancer drugs Anaesthetic drugs Antimicrobial drugs Stimulants Muscle relaxants Anticholinergics

Table 4. Conditions causing delirium in the elderly.

The addition of a drug that further depresses respiration could complicate the mental symptoms.

Advanced age is an important risk factor for delirium, particularly in patients who have become frail. In frail elderly patients, any medical illness has the potential to precipitate delirium. Indeed, altered state of consciousness is a typical presentation of acute myocardial infarction, dehydration with electrolyte imbalance, pneumonia or other infections in this age group.

For the primary care physician, an altered state of consciousness, particularly in an elderly patient, presents a diagnostic problem analogous to fever of unknown origin.

Neurological conditions causing dementia

Dementia can be caused by many other neurological conditions, some of which are extremely rare (Table 5). One must keep in mind that the dementia syndrome can have more than one aetiological basis in the older patient.

Differential diagnosis of dementia
Alzheimer's disease
Vascular dementias
Multi-infarct dementia
Binswanger's disease
Dementia with Lewy bodies
Diffuse Lewy body disease
Lewy body variant of AD
Parkinson's disease
Other dementias
Frontotemporal dementia
Creutzfeldt–Jakob disease
Progressive supranuclear palsy
Huntington's disease
Down's syndrome
Normal pressure hydrocephalus
Infection-related dementias
Alcoholism and drug abuse

Table 5. Differential diagnosis of dementia.

Vascular dementia

Besides AD (more than 60% of all dementias) the most frequent form appears to be vascular dementia (VaD; 10–20%). As they share many symptoms, it is not always easy to distinguish between those two forms. AD and VaD frequently appear in a mixed form, as do AD and dementia with Lewy bodies.

VaD encompasses instances where the pathology is associated with ischaemic, haemorrhagic and/or hypoxic–ischaemic cerebral lesions. The underlying risk factors for cerebrovascular disease (CVD) include hypertension, diabetes, coronary artery disease, atrial fibrillation, hyperlipidaemia, smoking and alcohol abuse.

The clinical picture of VaD usually includes abrupt deterioration in cognitive functions or fluctuating stepwise progression of cognitive defects (Table 6). Focal signs and symptoms are frequently present. Brain imaging – computed tomography (CT) and magnetic resonance imaging (MRI) (including diffusion weighted imaging) – would be likely to demonstrate cerebrovascular insults. Large-vessel lesions of the dominant hemisphere or bilateral large-vessel hemispheric strokes may suddenly produce VaD. Bilateral thalamic vascular

AD and VaD: diagnostic differences		
Feature	**VaD**	**AD**
Onset	Sudden or gradual	Gradual
Progression	In steps, fluctua-	Continuously
Gait	tions may be disturbed early	Normal until severe stage
CV conditions	Cardiovascular risk factors, previous stroke or transient ischaemic attacks	Less common (prevalent in mixed form)
Neurological	Focal deficits	Signs may not be present
Findings/imaging	Multiple infarcts	None but atrophy

Table 6. AD and VaD: diagnostic differences.

lesions, strokes in the association areas (parietal temporal, temporo-occipital territories) and bilateral anterior cerebral artery strokes are frequently associated with VaD. Progressive and extensive small-vessel disease with multiple lacunae may produce more gradual stepwise deterioration.

There are several features to help distinguish the two forms of dementia, AD and VaD, e.g. onset, disease progression or gait (Table 6).

There is also a relationship between AD and impaired supply of blood, glucose and oxygen to the brain. Cardiac disease can be an independent risk factor for AD. There is also active interest in the possibility of microvascular lesions in AD, perhaps related to cerebrovascular amyloidosis.

Binswanger's disease

Binswanger's disease (BD) is considered to be of vascular origin, related to chronic hypertension. Clinically, the picture is that of a multi-infarct dementia with the pathological changes greatest in the cerebral white matter, particularly in the territory of the long penetrating arteries. Clinical features are suggested by the picture of a subcortical dementia with gait apraxia, hyperreflexia and personality changes in a patient with risk factors for vascular diseases. Cognitive deficits can result from cerebral infarcts in strategic brain areas (with specific lesions to be found with neuroimaging techniques). BD patients show evidence of fluctuating dementia, with memory disorders in combination with a variety of focal motor impairments.

Dementia with Lewy bodies

This entity has previously been referred to as "diffuse Lewy body disease", "Lewy body variant of AD", "cortical Lewy body disease" or "senile dementia of the Lewy body type".

Lewy bodies are neuronal inclusion bodies consisting of neurofilament material, to be found in neuronal cytoplasm. The presence of Lewy bodies in the neocortex is the finding necessary to arrive at diagnosis. Lewy bodies are found most often in the temporal lobe, in the cingular gyrus, in the amygdala and in the insula.

The memory loss in patients with Lewy body dementia may be more subtle than in those with AD. The patients mostly exhibit rather spontaneously parkinsonian-type symptoms, hallucinations, delusions and disorders of executive function and show progressive illness leading to very severe dementia. The extrapyramidal/parkinsonian-type features may be mild.

Although clinically the diagnosis is being made more readily, one must await pathological confirmation.The patients clinically present with severe visual spatial impairment – which is picked up by clock drawings or by drawing figures, slowness in executive function with impaired judgement, visual hallucinations and some parkinsonian features.

The ApoE4 allele appears to be a major risk factor for Lewy body disease, as it is with AD.

Usually, patients with Lewy body dementia do not tolerate the older antipsychotic medications, which generate cholinergic and extrapyramidal side-effects.

Parkinson's disease

As many as 30% of elderly patients with Parkinson's disease (PD) develop dementia. Clinical and histopathological overlap between AD and PD is common.

Individuals with clear-cut clinical manifestations of PD and a progressive dementia who have Lewy bodies in the brain stem, plus the presence of sufficient senile plaques and neurofibrillary tangles to meet the diagnostic criteria for AD, are to be diagnosed with combined PD and AD.

Normal pressure hydrocephalus

Normal pressure hydrocephalus (NPH) or occult hydrocephalus may present with symptoms of memory loss, ataxia and apraxia of gait, as well as urinary incontinence. Changes in mental status occur as a result of impaired cerebrospinal fluid (CSF) flow. The 65-year-old female whose CT scan is shown in Figure 3A presented with such symptoms.

Isotope cisternography is utilized primarily for the demonstration of some types of hydrocephalus. Isotope is injected into the subarachnoid space in the lumbar region. Serial

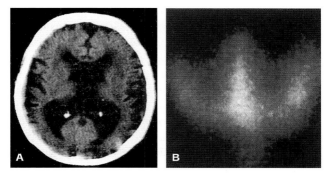

Figure 3. (A) CT brain scan of a 65-year-old female with progressive dementia, gait apraxia and ataxia, and urinary incontinence. Marked dilatation of the lateral and third ventricles is seen. (B) Nuclear cisternography of the same woman demonstrates penetration of the nucleotide into both the third and fourth ventricles, as well as into the markedly dilated lateral ventricles. Clinical and imaging findings were compatible with normal pressure hydrocephalus (NPH).

images are obtained to monitor the uptake, flow and absorption of the isotope within the ventricular system over a 72-hour period. The pattern of penetration and retention of isotope into the markedly dilated lateral ventricles characteristic of NPH is shown in Figure 3B.

There has been considerable discussion pertaining to shunting procedures once NPH has been demonstrated. In our experience, those who are identified early, before irreversible brain damage has occurred, may show gratifyingly beneficial results from surgical treatment.

Frontotemporal dementia

Frontotemporal dementia (FTD) is possibly the second most frequent degenerative cause of dementia. Alzheimer pathology is not present. FTD is considered to be a presenile dementia since patients may become symptomatic in their fifties and sixties. Three possible subtypes are based on where the pathological process appears to originate.

Primary progressive aphasia begins in the brain's *left hemisphere*, affecting language functions initially.

Patients with *right temporal variants* tend to experience earlier and more prominent changes in personality and may be mistaken for psychoses such as schizophrenia. These patients may suddenly begin exhibiting aggressive and other socially unacceptable behaviours.

The third type of FTD affects *both frontal lobes* initially. It occurs with and without Pick bodies, which are argyrophilic inclusions in neuronal cells. Only those FTD patients with these bodies are said to have Pick's disease, which may be inherited as an irregular autosomal dominant or recessive trait or may occur sporadically. These patients mainly begin to experience problems with organizing and planning. They may also show disinhibited behaviour and word-finding problems.

Huntington's disease

Huntington's disease (HD) may rarely occur late in life with chorea and dementia. It is inherited as an autosomal dominant trait through a trinucleotide expansion mutation in a gene, located on chromosome 4. Clinical features include changes in personality and deterioration in cognitive ability. Severe depressive symptoms may also develop.

Creutzfeldt–Jakob disease

A rapidly progressing, rare dementia with pyramidal, extrapyramidal and cerebellar signs, as well as myoclonus, would suggest the presence of Creutzfeldt–Jakob disease (CJD), which is caused by prions. The onset usually is in the sixth or seventh decade of life. Symptoms of irritability and unusual somatic sensations are common. Characteristic changes are present on the EEG with a periodic discharge pattern of 1–2 hertz (Hz). Familial forms have also been identified (Gerstmann–Straussler–Scheinker disease).

Harrington *et al.* (1986) demonstrated that the cerebrospinal fluid of CJD patients contains abnormal protein fractions. The amino acid sequence matched that found in a brain protein known as 14-3-3. A radioimmunoassay was developed and proved 14-3-3 to be a sensitive and relatively specific marker for prion diseases in humans and in animals.

Progressive supranuclear palsy

Dementia occurs in about 60–80% of patients with progressive supranuclear palsy (PSP), though it is not an obligate part of the syndrome that is accompanied by parkinsonism and ophthalmoparesis. Frontal lobe deficits are common in PSP, and are recognized with functional imaging techniques.

Dementia and Down's syndrome

The localization of the APP gene on chromosome 21q is utilized as an explanation of the finding that patients with Down's syndrome (trisomy 21) develop dementia with the classical neuropathological features of AD at the age of 30 years and slightly higher. Because of the characteristic features of Down's syndrome there should be no difficulty in differential diagnosis.

Infection-related dementias

Many neuropsychiatric manifestations of AIDS, including confusion, disorientation, memory loss, depression and agitation, as well as neuropathological findings, have been observed. Other subacute or chronic infectious diseases may cause memory loss and other symptoms of dementia. Among these are chronic fungal meningitis, viral encephalitis, CJD, neurosyphilis and early tuberculous meningitis.

Alcoholism and drug abuse

Many older persons with alcoholism or drug abuse are in denial, leading to under-diagnosis. Some AD patients compound the disease with sequelae from chronic alcoholism. Dementia in Wernicke–Korsakoff syndrome relates to alcoholism and nutritional deficiency. Heroin abusers who experienced coma from "overdose" reactions may develop dementia. Adverse reactions to hallucinogens may lead to permanent brain changes.

Clinical course and disease stages of AD

AD is a slowly progressive disease. The functional impairment and the severity of symptoms allow a basic distinction of disease stages, ranging from mild (stage I) to moderate (stage II) and to severe (stage III) (Table 7). Some authors add a fourth, quasi-terminal stage of so-called profound AD with very low or even untestable MMSE score. There is of course a preclinical presymptomatic phase, deeper knowledge of which is still lacking. Clearly, however, the pathology of the AD begins years before the first symptoms and functional impairments are manifest.

Symptom progression of Alzheimer's disease			
Function	**Stage I (mild)**	**Stage II (moderate)**	**Stage III (severe)**
Language	Anomia	Sensory aphasia	Severely impaired
Memory	Amnesia	Recent/remote	Untestable impairments
Abstraction	Impaired	Impaired	Untestable
Visuospatial	Mild to moderate impairment	Abnormal	Untestable
Behaviour	Indifferent, delusional	Indifferent, delusional	Agitated, stuporous, delusional
Gait	Normal	Wandering	Impaired
Posture	Normal	Normal	Flexed, bedridden
MMSE	30–21	20–11	10–0

Table 7. Symptom progression of Alzheimer's disease.

Recent findings in the literature suggest a pre-dementia stage associated with a high risk of progression to overt AD (10% per year), so-called mild cognitive impairment (MCI). The patients present with mild memory complaints but are still free from a decline in cognitive functioning. Light changes in personality may already be obvious.

Considering a theoretical time line from the onset of the pathological process in the brain with a gradually growing pathological burden that finally interferes with the functional status, there is a threshold at which the degree of neuropathological damage results in overt clinical dementia. By definition, this threshold is marked by the decline in functional capacity that interferes with the person's activities of daily living (ADL).

The earlier stages

The presymptomatic state is characterized as an insidious pathological process that takes place in the brain. The subtle, possibly resulting deficits can, however, be detected by thorough formal testing of cognitive performance. As the person approaches the threshold for clinical dementia, there may be signs of functional and cognitive deterioration, which can be caught by the MMSE and other dementia rating scales.

In the mild stage of AD, the memory impairment doubtlessly interferes with everyday activities. The handling of daily activities becomes more and more difficult, and the patient may appear as no longer reliable. Handling of finances causes problems and car driving begins to be risky, mainly because of loss of orientation and the increasing lack of understanding of the meaning of traffic signs. The first personality changes become obvious. Usually, the recognition that something bad and serious is going on causes anger and frustration in the patient, whose growing deficits are at the same time recognized and are often equalled by the frustration and anger of the family.

This is also the stage at which the amelioration of treatable components of the disorder may allow the (non-AD) patient to return temporarily to more normal functioning.

In the earlier stages, the neuropsychological impairments may be relatively selective. Chronic diseases of the brain tend to be asymmetric in onset. If the AD process affects the dominant (usually left) side of the brain first, then problems with language tend to be most evident early. In other patients, the non-dominant hemisphere (usually right) is involved more markedly in earlier stages. These patients tend to have problems organizing activities in space and a kind of flattening of expressed feelings. In some patients, the disease process first prominently affects areas of the brain subsuming emotion and organization of thought (limbic and/or frontal areas). In these patients, personality changes and psychoses could be particularly prominent (Figure 4).

The later stages

As the disease progresses, more and more of the brain becomes involved (the pathological burden grows further), until all of these functional domains become increasingly impaired. The patient then clearly shows global cognitive impairments. In the last phases, the patient depends on help and care for the simplest functions of existence, such as feeding, toileting and even mobility.

The rate of progression of AD is variable. Patients can go from health to terminal stages in about five to ten years. Others survive longer than 15 years. One reason for this might be the intensity and (emotional) quality of care.

Plateaus can be seen in the course of AD, lasting a year or more, as well as certain short-lived spontaneous improvements. Over time, however, the disease progresses mercilessly. At the end, the deterioration can take place rapidly. This may be due to the complete exhaustion of cerebral reserves or perhaps to an acceleration in the disease process itself.

The functional decline of a patient over the course of the disease can be outlined according to the activities of daily living that cause increasing difficulties. The following are examples. At the beginning there is the failure of keeping appointments and misplacing things (years 0–2); this phase is followed by problems with travelling alone and dressing (years 2–4).

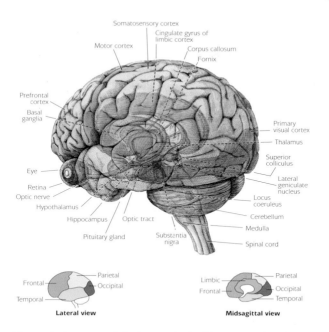

Figure 4. Anatomy of the human brain. The temporal and parietal lobes are particularly vulnerable for earliest dysfunction caused by the degenerative process of AD, corresponding with the early symptoms of the dementia. With permission from Carol Donner.

As the MMSE score decreases the level of dependence increases; the patient can no longer maintain hobbies and has difficulties with his personal hygiene (years 5–6/7). The loss of independent performance becomes complete in the last phase, with an MMSE score of under 10 (years 7–10) (Figure 5).

Patients with AD may have a life expectancy of as little as 3 years from diagnosis or they can live as long as 20 years from symptom onset. The average survival lies somewhere in between and reaches 8–10 years.

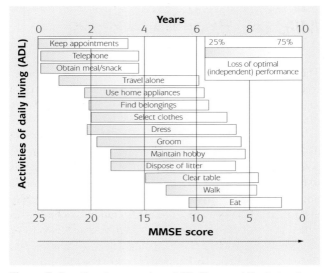

Figure 5. Functional progression of AD. The panel illustrates the correlation between activities of daily living (ADL) and the MMSE score over the years. Reproduced with permission from Galasko, D. (1998) An integrated approach to the management of Alzheimer's disease: assessment of cognition, function and behaviour. *Eur. J. Neurol.* **5** (suppl 4), S9–S17. Copyright © 1998 Blackwell Science Ltd.

Mild cognitive impairment

The concept of mild cognitive impairment (MCI) is a rather recent one, derived from the intensive search for reliable criteria for early diagnosis of AD. About 5–6% of the older population (65–79 years) meet the criteria for MCI.

MCI is considered to be a risk factor for the development of AD. And as more and more treatment options with the potential of modifying the course of the disease arise, it appears to be of critical importance to identify people at risk. This is not an easy task, because of the difficulty to clinically distinguish MCI from age-associated cognitive decline or so-called normal benign ageing. However, it now seems to be accepted that cognitive decline is not part of normal ageing. Even a mild decline may herald the onset of AD.

MCI can be considered as a precursor stage or even an early manifestation of clinical overt AD, characterized by isolated memory disturbances. There are usually no deficits in other cognitive domains at this stage of the beginning of impairment and there is no functional decline.

Case control studies indicate an increased conversion rate from MCI to AD with an average of about 10–12% or even 15% of cases per year. This contrasts with a conversion rate of 1–2% in the normal elderly population. The patients with MCI who are likely to develop AD in the near future present certain structural correlates that appear to be predictive. One of those is a (compared to normal age-matched controls) smaller hippocampal volume. Also, they appear to experience a more rapid atrophy of the hippocampus.

Though not yet fully established, there can be offered a list of criteria for diagnosing MCI in elderly patients that seems to be of some specificity (Table 8). When true memory impairment occurs in the absence of confounding conditions, emerging data indicate that progression of MCI to more overt dementia occurs predictably and is supported by neuropathological evidence of AD (Figure 6).

Proposed diagnostic criteria for MCI
Memory complaints
Memory function worse than in normal ageing
Absence of dementia
No further cognitive decline, normal functioning in ADL
Normal general cognitive function
Source: Petersen *et al.* (1999) *Arch. Neurol.* **56**, 303–308.

Table 8. Proposed diagnostic criteria for MCI.

Ageing	Early AD	Late AD
	Preclinical Very mild	
Cognitive normality	First clinical detection of dementia	Severe dementia
No plaques, or only patchy diffuse plaques in neocortex	Marked increase in neocortical amyloid deposition, including some neuritic plaques	Many neuritic plaques throughout cortex
Slow formation of tangles in limbic regions, none in neocortex	Increase in tangles, including some in neocortex	Many tangles in neocortex and hippocampus
None ⟶ Detectable		

Figure 6. Hypothetical sequence of clinico-pathological findings in ageing and AD. Reproduced with permission from Morris, J. (1999) Is Alzheimer's disease inevitable with age? *J. Clin. Invest.* **104** (9), 1171–1173. Copyright © 1999 American Society for Clinical Investigation.

There is growing evidence that vascular factors may contribute to the development of late-life cognitive impairment. A relationship with elevated systolic blood pressure has been found, as well as with high serum cholesterol levels, both at midlife. The precise mechanisms that cause the elevated risk of MCI remain unknown. Yet, there is a suggestion that the induction of atherosclerosis by chronic high blood pressure and hypercholesterolaemia combined with reduced arterial blood flow directly affects neurodegeneration relevant to AD and MCI (as prodromal stage for AD).

Long-standing hypercholesterolaemia may induce thickening of the intima and alterations in endothelial function in cerebrovascular arterioles and capillaries. These changes might impair brain metabolism. Cholesterol also exerts effects on the metabolism and production rate of APP.

The office-based work-up: clinical examination

The clinical examination and assessment of the patient is the cornerstone of the diagnostic approach. The main goal is the identification of the disease at an early stage.

The clinical diagnosis of AD can be made with great accuracy using ordinary clinical techniques available to physicians. Indeed, for primary care or family physicians, who know their patients rather well, the added work-up needed is limited. The diagnosis is much harder and requires a much more extensive evaluation when a new patient is seen who is confused and may be demented. It is even harder if there is no reliable informant who can provide a trustworthy history.

AD is, in spite of all recent findings, in the office of the primary care physician basically a diagnosis of exclusion. It depends on the presence of dementia with no other discernible cause to which the memory disorder can be attributed. The diagnosis of AD can be suspected even in the presence of another potentially dementing disorder, but it then cannot be made with confidence.

Patient history

An accurate history (anamnesis) is always critical. This is attained either by questioning the patient or through information given by the relative or caregiver.

Physical and neurological examination

Confusion can be the presenting sign of a wide variety of relatively acute medical and neurological conditions in the elderly. The evaluation, however conducted, needs to be careful and thorough. If the physician knows the patient, he should look for new signs. The new onset of focal weakness might indicate a superimposed stroke or even early signs of evolving subdural haematoma.

If the physician does not know the patient, then he should plan to focus even more intensively on potentially abnormal neurological exam findings.

Mental status testing

"Global Cognitive Impairment" means, in practice, that the patient has difficulties with memory and with at least two other areas (domains) of cognitive function. For the primary care physician, the Mini Mental State Examination (MMSE), developed by Folstein, Folstein and McHugh, provides a robust, simple, economic addition to the physician's ability to initially assess and follow patients with cognitive impairments. The MMSE is particularly useful for revealing deficits in patients, whose social skills are preserved and are skilfully used to disguise their mental impairments (Table 9).

The MMSE evaluates, albeit not in great depth, a variety of important functions, including short- and long-term memory, calculation, orientation, and constructional ability. Age-related norms are available. In ordinary use, a patient who scores less than 24 (of 30) is usually classified as having dementia or some other condition impairing cognitive function. A patient who scores 20 or less is likely to be clearly impaired, even if relatively mildly, in activities of daily life (ADL).

There is an educational curve in the MMSE. People who have a low level of school education consistently do worse than those with at least primary school education.

Clock drawing may provide a quick measure of cognitive function. The clinician or office staff member asks the patient for a free drawing of a clock. The accuracy of the drawing is a valid measure of the patient's cognitive state. Examples of healthy elderly controls and patients with dementia of varying severity are given in Figure 7.

Laboratory assessment

Laboratory tests are conducted to rule out possible reasons or conditions that could mimic or be responsible for memory problems or worsen a dementia. This means the laboratory assessment is targeted at identifying possible reversible causes. All patients with suggested AD should undergo comprehensive laboratory testing (Table 10).

A titre for Lyme disease may be appropriate in geographic regions, such as the northeast USA, where Lyme disease is

Mini Mental State Examination

	Score	Points
ORIENTATION		
1. What is the		
Year?	____	1
Season?	____	1
Date?	____	1
Day?	____	1
Month?	____	1
2. Where are we		
State?	____	1
County?	____	1
Town/city?	____	1
Floor?	____	1
Address/name of building?	____	1
REGISTRATION		
3. Name three objects, taking one second to say each. Then ask the patient all three after you have said them. Score first try. Repeat objects until all are learned.	____	3
ATTENTION AND CALCULATION		
4. Can you subtract 7 from 100, and then subtract 7 from the answer you get and keep subtracting 7 until I tell you to stop? (Stop after 5 answers.)	____	5
RECALL		
5. Ask for names of three objects learned in question 3. Give one point for each correct answer.	____	3
LANGUAGE		
6. Point to a pencil and a watch. Have the patient name them as you point.	____	2
7. Have the patient repeat "No ifs, ands, or buts."	____	1
8. Have the patient follow a three-stage command: "Take the paper in your right hand. Fold the paper in half. Put the paper on the floor."	____	3
9. Have the patient read and obey the following: "Close your eyes."	____	1
10. Have the patient write a sentence of his or her own choice. (The sentence should contain a subject and an object and should make sense. Ignore spelling errors when scoring.)	____	1
11. Here is a drawing. Please copy the drawing on the same paper. (Correct is the two five-sided figures intersect so that their juncture forms a four-sided figure and all angles in the five-sided figures are preserved.)	____	1

	TOTAL	30

Crum, R.M.; Anthony, J.C.; Bassett, S.S.; Folstein, M.F. (1993) Population-based norms for the Mini-Mental State Examination by age and educational level. *JAMA* **69**, 2420–2421.
Folstein, M.F.; Folstein, S.E.; McHugh, P.R. (1975) "Mini-Mental State": a practical method for grading the cognitive state of patients for the clinician. *J. Psychiat. Res.* **12**, 189–198.
Folstein, M.; Anthony, J.C.; Parhad, I. *et al.* (1985) *J. Am. Geriatr. Soc.* **33**, 228–235.

Table 9. Mini Mental State Examination (MMSE).

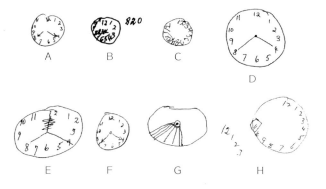

Figure 7. Clock drawing test; examples of the drawing by normal elderly controls and patients with dementia. Clocks A (MMSE 30), D (MMSE 29) and F (MMSE 30) were drawn by controls. Clocks B (MMSE 20), C (MMSE 19), G (MMSE 14) and H (MMSE 19) were drawn by patients with dementia. The patient who drew clock E (MMSE 29) showed only memory impairment on neuropsychological testing at the time of the drawing, but within 6 months of testing had deteriorated sufficiently to meet criteria for a diagnosis of probable AD.

Laboratory testing for AD
Urinalysis (optional: 24 hours for heavy metals, toxicology)
Complete blood count, sedimentation rate, ANA, C-reactive protein
Liver enzymes
Creatinine, BUN
Electrolytes, calcium, glucose
Vitamin B_{12}, folate
TSH, free thyroid index
Syphilis serology
HIV testing (consider even in the elderly)
Epstein–Barr viral titre
Lyme disease titre (in endemic areas)
ApoE genotyping (optional, in case of positive family history)

Table 10. Laboratory testing for AD.

endemic. Screening for syphilis and HIV titres should be considered. Recently, in some US retirement communities, a number of sexually promiscuous elderly persons have become HIV-positive.

If there is evidence for chronic fatigue, Epstein–Barr viral titre may be useful. Blood sedimentation rate, ANA or C-reactive protein enable the identification of patients with unrecognized medical disorders leading to cerebral damage, such as cerebral vasculitis. B_{12} levels should routinely be determined in elderly patients, as unrecognized B_{12} deficiency may produce significant neuropsychiatric symptoms. Hypothyroid or even "apathetic" forms of hyperthyroidism are to be considered.

Imaging techniques

Clinical diagnostic tools include brain imaging and cardiovascular tests. CT or MRI is now part of standard American practice, even though the yield of treatable illness is still low. Brain scans will detect subdural haematomas and tumours, and, along with isotope cisternography, may help identify the rare patient with normal pressure hydrocephalus who may respond well to brain-shunting procedures.

Single photon emission computed tomography (SPECT) is a procedure widely available nowadays. Multiple "punched out" lesions on a SPECT scan may help delineate the process of what was previously called multi-infarct dementia, today referred to as vascular dementia. The typical pattern early in AD is a decreased isotope uptake in the temporal/parietal areas bilaterally. In late stages of the disease, the changes become more widespread and severe.

Cardiological evaluation

Cardiological studies such as echocardiogram and Holter or event monitoring may raise suspicions of cardiogenic factors in inducing dementia in certain patients. It is very gratifying to see reversal of a dementing process in a person, whose myocardial neural conduction defect has been recognized and treated with a pacemaker implant, thereby restoring adequate brain vascular perfusion (Figure 8).

Follow-up

If the patient is indeed developing AD, follow-up evaluations will reveal gradual, progressive worsening of the neuropsychiatric symptoms detected.

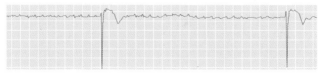

Figure 8. This ECG rhythm strip was recorded from a patient (89-year-old woman) with sick sinus node syndrome and atrial arrhythmias who demonstrated episodic and progressive confusion, which was misinterpreted as early dementia. A pacemaker was implanted, the cardiac rhythm normalized, and the mental symptoms cleared.

Neuropsychological tests for diagnosis, follow-up and measurement of therapeutic outcome

As part of the diagnosis there has to take place a basic screening of the patient's mental status. This is an essential feature of a dementia assessment and is best done by utilizing the Mini Mental State Examination (MMSE), developed by Marshal Folstein *et al.* It is important for the clinician to document means of estimating whether a patient's performance falls within age-appropriate norms.

The **MMSE** assesses in only 5–10 minutes the following cognitive domains: orientation, memory, attention, recall, language. The MMSE is widely used to measure the onset, the progression and the severity of AD, as well as the outcome of a therapeutic trial. The test has a range of 30 points, from normal (30) to severe impairment (0), and is to be performed by the patient himself. The average yearly change in patients with AD reaches 3 points.

The advantage of instruments such as the MMSE is also the possibility of predicting the future course. A bad score at baseline or a rapid fall in an unusually short period of time is certainly an unfavourable prognostic sign. On the other hand, early cognitive deterioration cannot always be easily caught by the MMSE, because of a ceiling effect in the relatively broad range of "normal", influenced by the level of education.

The cognitive assessment utilizing the **ADAS-cog** (Alzheimer's Disease Assessment Scale – cognitive subscale) may also be performed. This test is supposed to be more sophisticated and sensitive than the MMSE. It has a range of 70 points, from normal (0) to severe impairment (70). Among 11 items it includes the following cognitive domains: memory, language, orientation, simple tasks (praxis). The average yearly change in untreated patients with AD reaches 5–10 points.

A patient with mild to moderate AD shows a score of 15–25 on the ADAS-cog.

The ADAS-cog is helpful for the baseline assessment of the patient at diagnosis, to be able to observe the progression of the disease and a possible therapeutic outcome.

The Clinical Dementia Rating scale (**CDR**) can be utilized from the time of the clinical manifestation of the disease (rating 0.5). It provides (since it was expanded) a score range from 0 to 5 (terminal). The CDR determines the stage of AD by scoring six cognitive areas: memory, orientation, judgement and problem solving, community affairs, home and hobbies, and personal care. The information is derived from an interview with the patient and the caregiver. By the time a patient reaches score 1.0 on the CDR, there is no doubt about him having dementia. As pointed out, the CDR is not an instrument for early diagnosis of AD. At the time of score 0.5, 50% of the neurons in the entorhinal cortex might already be lost – though these patients are considered clinically as "normal".

Information on the progressive cognitive decline is also derived from the Global Deterioration Scale (**GDS**), developed by Barry Reisberg *et al.*, which consists of seven stages (1 = none, 7 = very severe).

The functional assessment addresses the patient's performance regarding the activities of daily living (ADL), including bathing, eating, dressing, transferring, toileting and continence. The so-called instrumental ADL (iADL) includes the use of the telephone, transportation, shopping, handling of finances and medication management. The less the ability of a patient to perform in the ADL, the more time is needed by the caregiver.

Outcome measures

The international requirements for the measurement of global outcome in studies with AD patients presently include four domains:

- cognition;
- global clinical changes, activities of daily living (ADL), quality of life (QoL);

- behaviour;
- resource utilization/health economics.

There are several rating scales that are to be used for the assessment; however, not all are evaluated and standardized. Major utilized rating scales are the ADAS-cog for the assessment of cognitive function, and Clinician's Interview-Based Impression of Change-plus care givers input (CIBIC-plus) for the measurement of global change (Table 11).

What, however, is clinically meaningful? An annual ADAS-cog deterioration of 8–11 points occurs in patients with moderately severe AD. There is some consensus that a pharmacological therapy in a clinical trial would be considered significant if the improvement on the ADAS-cog rating scale reaches at least –6 points (FDA Advisory Committee, 1989).

The measurement of global change utilizing **CIBIC-plus** is performed by the clinician and also requires the input of the caregiver. The score range is from 1 to 7: scores 1, 2 and 3 = improvement; score 4 = no change; scores 5, 6 and 7 = deterioration. CIBIC-plus measures the effect on global functioning, including cognition, functional stage and behaviour.

Standard outcome measures		
Rating scale	**Scoring**	**Assessments**
Cognitive function ADAS-cog	0–70 (low scores indicate better function)	Memory, attention, learning, orientation
Global change CIBIC-plus	1–7 (very much improved to very much worse)	Functional ability, cognitive performance and behaviour

ADAS-cog: Alzheimer's Disease Assessment Scale – cognitive subscale.
CIBIC-plus: Clinician's Interview-Based Impression of Change – plus caregiver input.

Table 11. Standard outcome measures.

Other frequently used test instruments for outcome measures in dementia include the Progressive Deterioration Scale (PDS) (functional ability, ADL), the Neuropsychiatric Inventory (NPI) (behaviour) and the Resource Utilization in Dementia (RUD) (caregiver time). The **PDS** measures the patient's function in ADL or quality of life and is rated by the caregiver. It is a questionnaire covering 29 items. The possible range is −100 to 100; positive differences indicate improvements.

In the case of a coexisting depression, the Hamilton Depression Scale (HamD) can be applied. The Geriatric Depression Scale in elderly AD patients can also be utilized.

Neuroimaging techniques in AD

Utilizing special techniques of structural and functional neuroimaging can help in assessing morphological, biochemical and physiological characteristics, and changes of evolving brain pathology. The modalities may not only aid the clinician in diagnosis, but contribute to planning the appropriate therapy and the follow-up of a demented person.

The formal role of imaging in establishing a clinical diagnosis, though, is to exclude possible causes of dementia other than AD, which may be identified through these techniques. The same holds true for excluding brain tumours (primary or metastatic) or other conditions, like subdural haematoma or brain abscesses. Hydrocephalus would also be recognized.

Cerebral white matter changes, periventricular and subcortical, on computed tomography (CT) or magnetic resonance imaging (MRI) should not be interpreted as presumptive evidence of dementia. Such patchy or confluent white matter alterations on MRI may reflect normal changes of ageing. Long-standing hypertension, for example, may also produce such lesions.

The differentiation between vascular dementia and other forms of dementia based simply upon white matter changes is doubtful, because such structural alterations are not limited to dementing illness.

Biochemical alterations can now be identified using MRI.

Functional imaging modalities may reveal characteristic regional bilateral temporal/parietal lobe or posterior cingulate deficits in patients with AD. These functional deficits, identified with positron emission tomography (PET), include regional deficits in glucose and oxygen metabolism, as well as in blood flow of the brain. Single photon emission computed tomography (SPECT) may reveal similar regional deficits in blood flow.

One major problem of neuroimaging remains the clear

differentiation between brain alterations associated with normal ("benign") ageing and changes as part of a pathological process. Jack and Petersen (in Scinto and Daffner, 2000) provide the explanation for a cognitive and morphological continuum: "Like cognition in the elderly", they state, "cerebral morphology exists in nature as a continuum, without categorizing into mild, moderate, or severe atrophy". However, it appears to be possible from the example of this continuum of cognition and morphology to explain the rather new concept of mild cognitive impairment – a stage between normal cognition/no brain atrophy, mild cognitive impairment/mild atrophy, dementia/ severe atrophy.

Computed tomography (CT)

Cerebral tissue is demonstrated moderately well, but CT does not give adequate contrasting images when tissue densities are similar, such as with white and grey brain matter. However, CT is superior to MRI in providing contrast between soft and hard tissues, such as bone versus cerebral tissue.

Many patients with a clinical diagnosis of AD appear to display more appreciable cortical atrophy on CT than expected for their age. However, the CT scan cannot be regarded as specific for the diagnosis of AD, since similar morphological changes throughout the cerebral cortex can also be seen in the absence of dementia.

Magnetic resonance imaging (MRI)

MRI is based upon nuclear spin density and two types of nuclear relaxation times (T_1 and T_2). Using this, the radiologist is able to identify different tissues. Tissue contrast with MRI is superior to that with CT. The intensity of lesions on T_1-weighted images is enhanced by contrast agents, thereby further documenting MRI as superior to CT in detection of subtle differences in brain tissue.

Like the CT scan, MRI gives a picture of the neuroanatomical structure and accurately reveals cerebral atrophy.

Hippocampal volume measurement

Volumetric studies with computer-enhanced MRI technology are being done to demonstrate both age-related changes and AD-related alterations in the medial temporal lobes and the limbic system. A decline with age can be found in patients with AD, which means hippocampal volumes of AD patients are smaller than those of age-matched controls.

As the AD progresses, significant volumetric changes may be seen in these susceptible regions. Therefore, such techniques are of help in assessing treatment effects on the course/progression of the disease. Such volumetric studies, however, would not be of help to the clinician in aiding in the early diagnosis of AD.

Positron emission tomography (PET)

PET today, still largely a research tool, permits the study of brain metabolism in living beings. The functional studies are mostly directed at evaluating cerebral blood flow and metabolism by measuring glucose or oxygen consumption. PET scanning can identify impairment in cortical blood flow (CBF) and glucose metabolism in the parietotemporal cortical areas in patients who are suspected of having AD even before the clinical findings are fully evident. Such information will be of increasing importance as future therapies directed at halting the disease progression become available.

Early differentiation between AD and frontotemporal dementia or dementia with Lewy bodies may also be possible via PET scanning.

Single photon emission computed tomography (SPECT)

SPECT provides estimates of cerebral perfusion, but unlike PET, it does not inform about glucose metabolism. SPECT is less sensitive in detecting early AD than PET scanning. Nonetheless, SPECT provides a unique approach to studying the function of the brain in patients with neuropsychiatric disorders. SPECT imaging is currently available in most large hospitals; the method is significantly cheaper than PET.

Most SPECT studies are designed to measure regional cerebral blood flow (rCBF). The predominant findings of bilateral, posterior temporal and parietal perfusion defects in a patient with memory disorder or other cognitive abnormality are highly predictive of AD. The observed reduced tracer uptake (gamma-emitting isotopes) is most likely related to diminished rCBF, decreased cortical thickness and loss of neurons within the affected areas. The severe bilateral perfusion defects seen on SPECT scan slices in a patient with advanced AD are shown in Figure 9.

In patients with vascular dementia, brain SPECT and diffusion-weighted MR imaging is superior to CT scanning in detecting very recent ischaemic events and lesions (Figure 10).

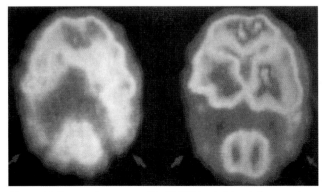

Figure 9. Severe, late-stage AD. SPECT brain blood-flow study shown in two slices, demonstrating temporoparietal and generalized cerebral functional impairment.

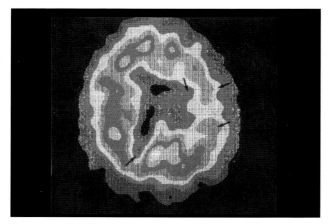

Figure 10. SPECT brain blood-flow study (using Tc-99m radiopharmaceutical) of a 77-year-old male. Generalized hypoperfusion is seen in the left cerebral hemisphere. Focal perfusion defects are also seen within the left basal ganglia and right occipital regions. This pattern of perfusion defects is characteristic of multiple cerebral infarctions, clinically consistent in this patient with vascular dementia.

Common medical problems in patients with AD

Because of their increasing disabilities resulting from the gradual decline in cognitive and functional capacity, patients with AD are prone to various medical problems, listed in Table 12. Effective management of the disease has to take these conditions into account.

In this context, the ethical dilemma has to be addressed, as effective therapy of the additional medical problems might result in a prolongation of life. Of special concern are the ethical issues surrounding physician or family insistence on inserting percutaneous feeding gastrostomies (PEG tubes). So the question of how aggressively a concomitant disease should be treated will always arise, particularly in the later stage of the disease. To resolve this dilemma, the physician should look for good communication with the caregiver, the family or the legal representative of the patient, whose potential will should be respected. Additionally, it would be wise to consult available national and/or international guidelines that address this specific topic.

Common medical problems in AD

- Falls and fractures
- Incontinence (urinary/faecal)
- Malnutrition with generalized muscle wasting
- Immobilization with contractures and rigidity
- Infections (urinary sepsis, pneumonia, decubitus ulcers with secondary infections)
- Cardiac arrhythmias, hypotension, congestive heart failure, stroke
- Delirium and seizures

Table 12. Common medical problems in AD.

Depression and dementia

One of the clinical challenges lies in the differentiation between dementia and depression. It is of major importance to diagnose the patient with depression, because this condition is treatable and is not associated with the bad prognosis.

Depression can be the first symptom of a developing dementing illness and is considered to be a risk factor for AD. At least one-third of all patients with AD will suffer from depressive symptoms at some stage of their disease.

There are several features which make a clear distinction between depression and dementia possible (Table 13).

Distinction between depression and AD		
Feature	**Depression**	**AD**
Onset/duration	Rapid, short	Gradual, long
Mood	Depressed	Irritable (early), apathetic (later)
Memory	Impairment of short- and long-term memory	Impairment of recent memory (early/moderate)
Orientation	Not impaired	Impaired
Clock drawing	Not impaired	Impaired

Table 13. Distinction between depression and AD.

Diagnostic biomarkers for AD

The ideal biomarker for the confirmation of AD should be able to detect a fundamental feature of the (neuro)pathological process, and this with as high a specificity and sensitivity as possible. It should be validated in AD, standardized, reproducible, non-invasive, simple to perform, and of course inexpensive.

There is no question that for early-onset familial AD (FAD) the search for mutations of the three candidate genes appears to be appropriate. The picture is different regarding late-onset and sporadic cases. Here, only the genetic detection of the ApoE4 allele serves to confirm the clinical diagnosis. The search for genetic abnormalities, however, should be limited to probands and families with a pattern of FAD.

"Among the other proposed molecular and biochemical markers for sporadic AD, cerebrospinal fluid assay showing low levels of Abeta42 and high levels of tau comes closest to fulfilling criteria for a useful biomarker", state the authors of the Consensus Report of the Working Group on Molecular and Biochemical Markers of Alzheimer's Disease (1998).

A series of biomarkers have been tried in AD; most of them tend to reflect the presently recognized neuropathological alterations in the brain of patients with AD, such as:
- amyloid protein derivatives in blood and cerebrospinal fluid (CSF);
- beta-amyloid peptide 42;
- beta-amyloid in plasma;
- beta-amyloid in urine;
- tau levels in CSF;
- neuronal thread proteins (NTPs) in CSF;
- CSF neurotransmitters and neurotransmitter metabolites.

All these tests can be considered promising, but the diagnostic utility is still limited. Further studies are required, including those with a combination approach.

The combination of the markers for the measurement of tau protein and beta-amyloid in the CSF, for example, appears rather successful. Beta-amyloid is a free-floating protein in the CSF. Its accumulation in the brain of AD patients with the formation of plaques is well known. This then leads to a reduction of beta-amyloid in the CSF. Abnormally phosphorylated tau protein is the main component of neurofibrillary tangles, also part of the brain pathology (Figure 11). The cellular destruction in AD causes a release of tau protein into the extracellular fluid, thereby increasing the CSF tau concentration. It is suggested, based on a number of studies, that elevated levels of tau and low levels of beta-amyloid in the CSF are diagnostic of AD.

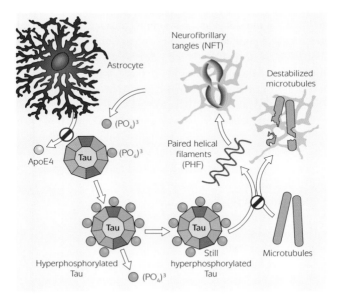

Figure 11. Pathophysiology of tau in AD with ApoE4. Figure courtesy of Athena Diagnostics.

Several tests are currently commercially available, such as Admark® Tau/Abeta42 CSF (correlates levels of tau protein and beta-amyloid peptide in the CSF), and Admark® Pofile (for the detection of ApoE alleles 2, 3 and 4, and levels of tau protein and beta-amyloid. Others include Innotest® beta-amyloid (1–42) and Innotest® hTau Ag, enzyme immunoassays for the detection of human beta-amyloid and human tau antigens in the CSF. Both are propagated for use in early diagnosis (even before the onset of clinical symptoms).

There is a large group of biochemical markers based on the detection of presumed specific systemic alterations in patients with AD; all of them lack sufficient specificity, and they are not considered useful as reliable biochemical markers. The group includes the skin test for beta-amyloid in circulating blood, the test of olfactory perception, fibroblast alterations, test of increased platelet membrane fluidity, demonstration of an elevation of iron-binding protein p97, and the tropicamide eye test for pupil dilatation.

Neuropathological findings in AD

The cause of AD is still not known, and the diagnosis is possible only post-mortem. The pathological picture of the brain of an AD patient at autopsy reveals massive brain atrophy and considerable loss of neurons and synapses. Two further typical findings include the presence of neuritic ("senile") plaques and neurofibrillary tangles (NFTs). There are also signs of astrocyte and microglial proliferation. The overall brain volume and weight is usually reduced in AD.

Other pathologies (of presumably minor importance) include the presence of neuropil threads (NTs) in the brain, which are considered an extension of the cytoskeletal pathology of AD. Further findings include granulovacuolar degeneration in pyramidal neurons of Ammon's horn of the hippocampus, Hirano bodies in or adjacent to pyramidal cells, and amyloid (congophilic) angiopathy in leptomeningial and cortical vessels in the cerebral cortex.

Senile plaques and amyloid

The senile plaque is a complex structure found in the neuropil that consists of a core of amyloid (formed from beta-amyloid protein), abnormal neurites and glial cells. The plaques occur in various types (diffuse or compact), and are distinguishable by electron microscopy. The presence of dystrophic neurites characterizes the neuritic plaque. Amyloid seems first to be deposited as diffuse, then later as neuritic plaques, representing a higher grade of degeneration (Figure 12A, B).

Amyloid has a key role in AD – in the absence of amyloid plaques the diagnosis of AD is not made, even if other features suggest the dementia. The small amyloid fragment in AD – beta-amyloid, consisting of 1–44 amino acids – arises from the much larger transmembrane molecule of amyloid precursor protein (APP). The APP gene, located on the long arm of chromosome 21, is its promoter. The function of APP has not

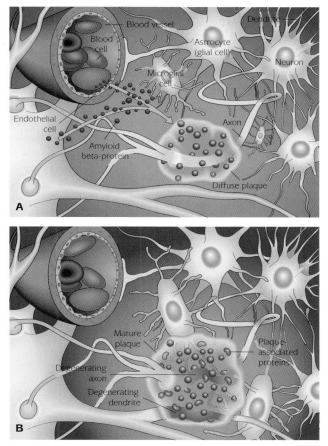

Figure 12. The role of beta-amyloid in causing AD is illustrated according to one hypothesis. (A) Beta-amyloid protein, which may be released by neurons, by glial cells or by cells in the circulatory system, accumulates in the nervous system as innumerable diffuse plaques. (B) The beta-protein, various glial cells and other proteins that become embedded in the plaque matrix as it matures may then gradually cause nearby neurons to degenerate. With permission from Toma Narashima and Dennis J. Selkoe.

yet been explained. Hypotheses include its role as a cell-adhesion molecule.

The metabolism of APP includes fragmentation (or cutting) of the large molecule by the enzyme alpha-secretase at the site of the neuronal membrane, resulting in a long and soluble extracellular fragment. In AD, two other enzymes (beta- and gamma-secretase) cut the APP molecule at different sites (Figure 13). The result of this mechanism is the production of the beta-amyloid fragment that is deposited in amyloid plaques. Direct inhibition of these secretases therefore appears to be a suitable future option for prevention and therapy of AD.

Amyloid is supposed to be toxic to brain cells and provokes an inflammatory reaction, followed by injuries. The inflammatory process, especially in the region of the neuritic plaque, is today the focus of greater attention, as it might perhaps open up future therapeutic pathways. The cascade of events, involving astrocyte-derived activated glial cells, oxidative stress resulting in free radical formation, disturbance of calcium homeostasis and mitochondrial membrane disruption, is somehow better understood (though far from being fully explained) in this way (Figure 14).

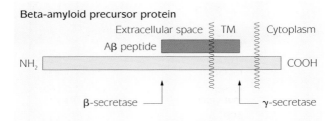

Figure 13. Proteolytic cleavages of amyloid precursor protein (APP) that produce beta-amyloid. Reproduced with permission from Selkoe, D.J. *et al.* (2000) The origins of Alzheimer disease. Editorial. *JAMA* **283** (12), 1615–1617. Copyright © 2000 American Medical Association.

Researchers today clearly state pathophysiological interactions among biochemical, environmental, genetic and inflammatory influences, leading to the characteristic pathology in AD with neuronal cell death.

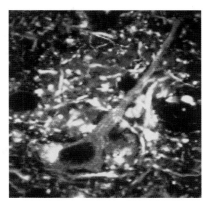

Figure 14. Laser scanning confocal microscopy of the lesions in AD. Plaque double immuno-labelled with an antibody against amyloid (red) and neuro filament (green) shows a neuron and its processes trapped in the midst of the amyloid mass. Reproduced with permission from Terry, R.D.; Katzman, R.; Bick, K.L. (1996) *Alzheimer's Disease*. New York: Lippincott-Raven. Copyright © 1996 Lippincott, Williams & Wilkins.

Genetic alterations and their pathological effects in AD			
Chromosome	**Gene product**	**Age of onset**	**Effect**
14	Presenilin 1 mutations	Early	Increased production of beta-amyloid
1	Presenilin 2 mutations	Early	Increased production of beta-amyloid
21	APP mutations	Early	Overproduction of beta-amyloid
19	ApoE4 polymorphism	Late	Increased deposition of beta-amyloid plaques, as well as vascular deposits

Table 14. Genetic alterations and their pathological effects in AD.

It is worth mentioning that the prominent pathological findings can be caused by genetic alterations (Table 14).

Neurofibrillary tangles

The neurofibrillary tangles (NFTs) are intraneuronal structures, which are composed of an altered microtubule-associated protein (MAP) called tau or tau protein. Tau is extensively cross-linked and phosphorylated, producing a highly insoluble protein with the structure of a paired helical filament. The mechanism that causes the alteration of tau is not yet known. The finding, however, is not specific for AD, as up to 80% of the normal elderly population will also develop NFTs in the entorhinal cortical regions by the age of 80 years and above. However, there seems to be a correlation of the number of NFTs with the severity of the disease. Therefore, prevention of their formation is one therapeutic goal.

NFTs are found particularly within the cortex, but also in other brain regions. In the cortex, the highest density of NFTs has been observed in limbic and paralimbic regions, such as the hippocampus and entorhinal cortex. A strong relationship between the density of NFTs and the severity of the dementia has been suggested.

Where do the structural changes in the brain of AD patients take place? Cortical neuron loss can be found in the following areas: amygdala, hippocampus, entorhinal cortex, nucleus basalis of Meynert, locus coeruleus. Neuropil and cellular disruption becomes prominent as a result of: formation of neuritic plaques and NFTs, amyloid deposition, synapse loss, oxidative stress. The dysfunction of these brain cells is associated with clinical findings.

Current therapies for AD

Currently no cure exists for patients with AD, and until recently there was no symptomatic therapy available for the primary deficits of AD, that is, memory disorders and cognitive decline.

All pharmacological attempts to treat AD culminate in the goal of preserving or improving cognitive function and to delay the progression of the disease into late stages for as long as possible. An appropriate management of the disease with currently available agents can stabilize the disease for a certain period of time, improve cognition, reduce behavioural disturbances, and thus delay the need for institutionalization.

The currently available therapeutic options for AD can be roughly divided into non-specific and specific pharmacological approaches. Most of the non-specific agents lack a thorough evaluation in AD; some of them have to be considered as obsolete. The criteria of evidence-based medicine are so far only met by the new acetylcholinesterase inhibitors (AChEIs), which have been carefully studied in clinical trials of sufficient duration and using adequate numbers of patients. Also thoroughly studied in AD is an extract of *Ginkgo biloba*.

Non-specific and non- or not-yet-proven agents

Neurotropic or nootropic agents such as **piracetam** and pyritinol have frequently been tried in AD and other forms of dementia, but there is overall little convincing evidence of any efficacy. The same holds true for drugs with vasodilator activity. Ergot derivatives were originally given to AD patients because they were thought to be peripheral and cerebral vasodilators. Agents such as **nicergoline** and **co-dergocrine mesylate** have been most commonly used. Their potential effectiveness, however, is now attributed to their action as metabolic enhancers or nootropic agents. More recent well-controlled studies found no benefit and their place in the therapy of AD has still to be established.

Calcium-channel blockers such as nimodipine have more recently been studied in patients with AD. The proclaimed mechanism is one of preventing calcium overload, particularly in aged ischaemic or otherwise damaged neurons. One of the mechanisms of cell loss in AD may involve an influx of calcium that causes neuronal dysfunction and/or neuronal death. By influencing neurotransmitter balance and by preventing excessive elevation of intracellular neuronal calcium levels, nimodipine or other calcium-channel blockers might be expected to prolong cell survival and improve cell function. Until now, however, no studies are available to prove this hypothesis, and the agents have to be considered non-specific and of no proven benefit.

Antioxidant and protective strategies

Propentofylline, a xanthine derivative with a proclaimed neuroprotective effect on astrocyte-derived glial cells, has been studied in AD and vascular dementia – without convincing evidence of successful treatment or benefit having been shown.

Numerous neurotransmitter deficiencies have been observed in patients with AD. However, the most consistent defect correlating with the severity of the condition is represented by reduced choline acetyltransferase activity, leading to reduced synthesis of acetylcholine. Different methods have been tried to increase the levels of acetylcholine in the brain. These attempts include the use and administration of **acetylcholine precursors**, cholinergic agonists, cholinesterase inhibitors and enhancers of acetylcholine release.

Treatments using precursors of acetylcholine such as **lecithine** or **choline** alone are not considered to produce useful improvements.

The books concerning the effects of selegiline, a selective **monoamine oxidase (MAO) inhibitor** with antioxidant potential, are not yet closed. Favourable results have been documented in short-term studies, but have not yet been confirmed in long-term-studies. The evaluation of **selegiline** and other MAO inhibitors was led by the finding that MAO type B activity is increased in patients with AD. Inhibition of this enzyme may provide a neuroprotective effect by scavenging the excess of free radicals that are toxic to nerve cells. Further clinical studies with selegiline, which exerts proven efficacy in Parkinson's disease, are under way.

Clinical trials with AD patients have been done to examine the possible benefits of the combination of selegiline and **vitamin E**. Either drug alone appeared to slow progression of the disease. The combination of both, however, did not cause additional improvement. Further studies testing the efficacy of vitamin E for preventing the transition from mild cognitive impairment (MCI) to the AD syndrome are under way.

Lazabemide is also a highly selective, reversible inhibitor of MAO-B. Preclinical data suggested efficacy. Initial clinical trials did not demonstrate efficacy and no further studies are being conducted.

Idebenone, a benzoquinone derivative, showed some benefit in the treatment of mental impairment associated with cerebrovascular disorders. The agent may exert its cytoprotective effects through an antioxidant mechanism. It protects against glutamate- and beta-amyloid-induced neurotoxicity in neuronal cell cultures. Clinical trials in AD patients did not show treatment efficacy.

Anti-inflammatory agents are being tried in AD, as the disease lesions are characterized by the presence of numerous inflammatory proteins. The extent by which inflammation contributes to the neurodegenerative process, however, is an open question. The available studies in AD are of limited value and statistical significance because of small size and insufficient design. However, the data suggest that anti-inflammatory agents might exert protective effects against AD, but only in low doses.

The major known effects of low-dose aspirin and other non-steroidal anti-inflammatory agents (NSAIDs) are on blood vessels and platelets with inhibition of cyclo-oxygenase. This enzyme happens to be a major tissue oxidant, converting the oxygen in haemoglobin to superoxide radicals. As platelets are the primary source of beta-amyloid in the blood, NSAIDs may directly reduce the amount of circulating beta-amyloid derived from platelets. Under these circumstances anti-inflammatory drugs, if effective, would be considered as preventive therapies for AD. However, as yet there is no convincing scientific evidence that anti-inflammatory agents are of benefit in the treatment of established AD.

Oestrogen, like other steroid sexual hormones, is supposed to have neuroprotective effects and it can induce antioxidant activity. Therefore, it may have a role in cognitive function (maintaining brain function) and neurodegeneration. The mechanism may be cholinergic stimulation via a neurotrophic effect on cholinergic neurons. Oestrogen can elevate the levels of the acetylcholine-synthesizing protein choline acetyltransferase (ChAT).

Oestrogens may also play a role in the processing of beta-amyloid precursor protein (APP) toward a non-amyloidogenic fragment. The hormone could thus reduce beta-amyloid production and its toxicity. This could explain the finding of a lower incidence of AD in postmenopausal women under hormone replacement therapy (HRT). However, the role of oestrogen in the prevention and treatment of AD remains to be determined. A large multicentre clinical trial to evaluate the effect of oestrogen in preventing AD or delaying its onset is currently under way in women 65 years of age or above who have had first degree relatives with AD.

Statins (hydroxy-methyl-glutaryl-coenzyme A reductase inhibitors) are lipid-lowering drugs, used in patients with lipid disorders (hypercholesterolaemia) or cardiovascular disease to inhibit synthesis of cholesterol. They are currently under evaluation.

The rationale behind this evaluation includes the finding of significantly higher levels of total and low-density lipoprotein (LDL) cholesterol in AD patients compared to non-demented persons. There is a relationship among levels of cholesterol and levels of the cholesterol-carrying protein apolipoprotein E (ApoE). It is also known that decreased levels of cholesterol in the diet will decrease the concentrations of beta-amyloid in the blood and decrease the levels of ApoE (and vice versa). Lowering cholesterol with statins therefore might decrease the total amount of beta-amyloid in the brain. Epidemiological data suggest a lower prevalence of AD in patients who take statins for cardiovascular-directed reasons.

Specific therapeutic agents

In view of the availability of well-designed clinical trials in AD only memantine, an extract of *Ginkgo biloba* (with reservations, however), and several third generation acetylcholinesterase inhibitors (AChEIs) can be regarded as rather specific palliative therapeutic agents.

Memantine, a derivative of amantadine, is a non-competitive blocker of *N*-methyl-D-aspartate (NMDA) receptor channels and a modulator of glutamatergic neurotransmission. NMDA receptor mechanisms have been linked to information coding by hippocampal neurons. Memantine is used in the treatment of Parkinson's disease, as well as brain injuries and dementia. It is approved for treatment of AD in parts of Europe.

It has been hypothesized that a non-competitive NMDA antagonist may have a beneficial effect on the course of AD in a symptomatic and neuroprotective way. Initial controlled clinical trials in AD have shown improvements of cognitive disturbances, drive, motivation and enhancement of motor functions. Further large-scale trials to confirm long-term efficacy and tolerability are under way for care-dependent patients in advanced stages of AD. One trial compares memantine with placebo. Another trial compares the effects of memantine or placebo on patients who had already been on a stable dose of donepezil prior to the study.

Ginkgo biloba extract EGb 761 produced certain improvement of cognitive functions in some patients with AD. However, if there is any, then the effect in older people with mild to moderate dementia is significantly smaller than the benefit of current AChEIs. The results of the recent clinical trials with EGb 761 are not at all consistent. Ginkgo is believed to exert a vasoregulatory action, which protects blood vessels and various tissues, and might explain its use in managing cerebral insufficiency states and neurosensory disturbances (among others). It is further supposed to exert cognition-enhancing and stress-alleviating actions. Finally, a gene-regulatory action is claimed. A primary prevention trial with EGb 761 is under way.

Acetylcholinesterase inhibitors (AChEIs)

The most significant improvement of cognitive symptoms thus far has resulted from the use of centrally active cholinergic agents, which inhibit the degradation of acetylcholine by the enzyme acetylcholinesterase. Cholinergic therapy can slow down the progression of AD but not cure the disease.

The prototype of the first generation of such agents is **physostigmine**, first used in short-duration AD trials in the early 1980s. Physostigmine retards deterioration. The compound does, however, exert unfavourable cholinergic side-effects. One derivative of physostigmine is **eptastigmine** (second generation), which shows good cholinergic tolerability but some degree of hepatic toxicity. Neither physostigmine nor eptastigmine are currently under further testing.

Metrifonate has been used for decades for the (short-term) treatment of schistosomiasis. It is an organophosphorous compound that is transformed into a long-acting inhibitor of acetylcholinesterase after oral administration. The agent was well tolerated and showed beneficial effects on memory, cognitive function and ADLs in a large number of patients with AD, including follow-up for more than 4 years. Then, however, safety problems were recognized and the further evaluation of the compound in AD was discontinued in 1999.

Velnacrine maleate is a primary degradation product of tacrine, which produced a relatively high initial (two-thirds of patients) response rate, as well as a rather high sustained response rate (40–50%) in patients with AD. The main problem was frequent adverse events with elevated liver enzymes and gastrointestinal cholinergic effects. It is no longer being tested.

The administration of AChEIs is based on the so-called cholinergic hypothesis. This pathology-based hypothesis led to the first rational approach to treatment of AD. The principle is straightforward – increase the level of acetylcholine in the brain to compensate for the decrease of this neurotransmitter found in AD. Among the early neuropathological findings was the observation that there was a severe neuronal loss in the nucleus basalis of Meynert. This nucleus sends projections to many areas of the cortex, particularly the frontal, parietal and hippocampal regions (Figure 15). Acetylcholine is the primary neurotransmitter of these neurons. A number of animal studies indicated that cholinergic function was vital to memory function and learning ability.

Acetylcholinesterase (AChE) activity is predominant in the healthy brain, while butyrylcholinesterase (BuChE) seems to have only a minor role in normal cholinergic transmission.

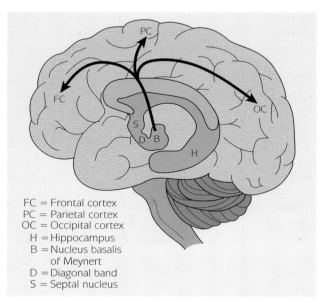

FC = Frontal cortex
PC = Parietal cortex
OC = Occipital cortex
 H = Hippocampus
 B = Nucleus basalis
       of Meynert
 D = Diagonal band
 S = Septal nucleus

Figure 15. Cortical cholinergic systems in the brain: forebrain cholinergic nuclei and their projections in different brain areas, related to the pathology of AD.

However, BuChE is significantly increased in the hippocampus and the cerebral cortex of patients with AD. BuChE also breaks down acetylcholine. The presumed additional inhibition of BuChE may therefore be of therapeutic benefit.

The new observation indicates that AChEIs and muscarinic agonists might be able to enhance the release of non-amyloidogenic-soluble derivatives of APP and possibly slow down the formation of amyloidogenic compounds in the brain. With this effect on APP metabolism, they would exert an anti-deterioration and protective effect.

Four AChEIs of the third generation are now approved for symptomatic therapy of AD: tacrine, donepezil, rivastigmine and galantamine. The first approved AChEI was **tacrine**. In

Dosage and administration of commonly used AChEIs			
Strategy	**Donepezil**	**Rivastigmine**	**Galantamine**
Dosing	Once daily	Twice daily	Twice daily
Starting dose (mg/day)	5	3	8
Lowest effective dose (mg/day)	5	6	16
Maximum dose (mg/day)	10	12	24
Dose increase	Increase to 10 mg/day after 4–6 weeks	Increase to 6 mg/day after 2 weeks; increases to 9 and 12 mg/day may be attempted after 2 weeks at previous dose	Increase to 16 mg/day after a minimum of 4 weeks; a further increase to 24 mg/day may be attempted after 4 weeks at previous dose

Table 15. Dosage and administration of commonly used AChEIs.

studies with AD patients, tacrine produced improvements in cognition and significant delays in the progression of deficits. The hepatic side-effect profile, however, made this agent rather problematic. Today, tacrine is considered obsolete.

Donepezil, a piperidine-based compound, is one of the modern highly selective, reversible AChEIs, marketed in 1997. The agent is now being widely utilized for the treatment of patients with mild to moderately severe AD. The lack of hepatic toxicity permits freedom from liver function monitoring. Donepezil exerts statistically significant efficacy over the long term in various measurements (MMSE, ADAS-cog, Quality of Life, QoL). The tolerability of this agent is good; one advantage is the once daily administration (Table 15).

The results of a 30-week controlled trial of 473 patients with mild to moderate AD are shown in Figure 16. Patients were randomized to either donepezil (5 or 10 mg) or placebo. The 24-week double-blind phase was followed by a 6-week single-blind

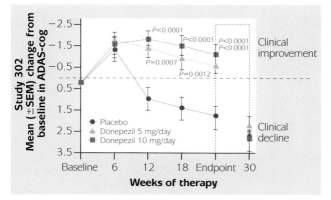

Figure 16. Efficacy of donepezil over a treatment period of 30 weeks, as measured with the ADAS-cog. Reproduced with permission from Rogers, S.L. *et al.* (1998) A 24-week, double-blind, placebo-controlled trial of donepezil in patients with Alzheimer's disease. *Neurology* **50,** 136–145. Copyright © 1998 Lippincott, Williams & Wilkins.

placebo washout phase. Statistically significant benefits in cognitive function as evaluated with the ADAS-cog with both dosages of donepezil were achieved (4.6 points over placebo for the high dose).

Winblad et al. (2001) reported a 1 year randomized study of donepezil versus placebo in patients with mild to moderate AD. The data demonstrated significant long-term benefits of donepezil administration over placebo on global assessment, cognition and ADL. Another double-blind placebo-controlled study (Mohs et al. 2001) has shown that treatment with donepezil for 1 year was associated with a 38% reduction in the risk of functional decline compared with placebo (Figure 17).

Additional studies are being conducted in patients with severe AD, vascular dementia, Lewy body dementia and in 18–35-year-old patients with trisomy 21 (Down's syndrome).

Rivastigmine is a dose-dependent pseudo-irreversible carbamate-selective inhibitor of AChE. The agent shows highly

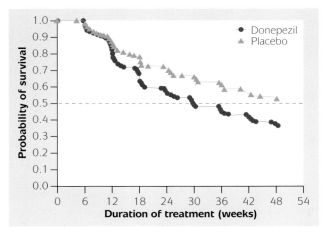

Figure 17. Kaplan–Meier survival estimates of time to clinically evident functional decline (by investigator, intent-to-treat population). Reproduced with permission from Mohs, R. C. *et al.* (2001) A 1-year, placebo-controlled preservation of function survival study of donepezil in AD patients. *Neurology* **57,** 481–488. Copyright © 2001 Lippincott, Williams & Wilkins.

selective binding and inactivation without hepatic microsomal inactivation. Similar improvements to donepezil are seen in cognition, ADL and global function. Behavioural symptoms may improve under this therapy. The tolerability can be impaired through unpleasant yet not severe cholinergic side-effects, especially gastrointestinal problems. Administration is twice a day, with initial dose titration necessary.

The efficacy of rivastigmine was documented in a 26-week double-blind controlled study with a total of 699 patients with mild to moderately severe probable AD. The patients were randomized to 6–12 mg/day rivastigmine, 1–4 mg/day rivastigmine, or placebo (Figure 18).

Statistically significant effects on cognition (compared to the patients under placebo, who continuously deteriorated) were achieved in the group of patients under the higher dose of rivastigmine. The difference on the ADAS-cog score over placebo was documented as 4.94 points over placebo (P < 0.05; high

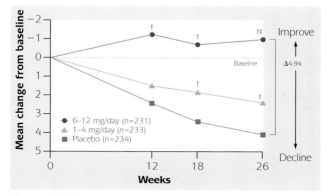

Figure 18. Efficacy of rivastigmine on cognition, as measured with the ADAS-cog over 26 weeks of therapy. †P < 0.05 vs placebo. ‡P < 0.05 vs rivastigmine (1–4 mg/day). Reproduced with permission from Corey-Bloom, J. *et al*. (1998) A randomized trial evaluating the efficacy and safety of ENA 713 (rivastigmine tartrate), a new acetylcholinesterase inhibitor, in patients with mild to moderately severe Alzheimer's disease. *Int. J. Geriatr. Psychopharmacol.* **1,** 55–65. Copyright © 1998 Nature Publishing Group.

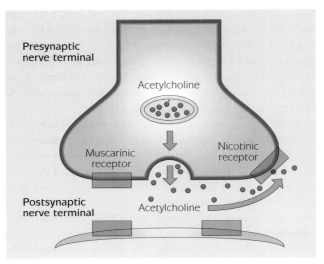

Figure 19. Pre- and postsynaptic nicotinic receptor sites for acetylcholine (ACh); delayed breakdown of ACh by AChEIs can result in continued activation of the presynaptic neuron. Figure courtesy of Edson X. Albuquerque, MD, PhD.

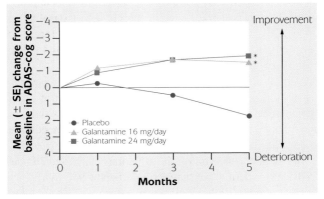

Figure 20. Efficacy of galantamine on cognition, as measured with the ADAS-cog over 20 weeks of therapy. *$P < 0.001$ vs placebo. Reproduced with permission from Tariot, P.N. *et al.* (2000) A 5-month, randomized, placebo-controlled trial of galantamine in AD. *Neurology* **54**, 2269–2276. Copyright © 2000 Lippincott, Williams & Wilkins.

dose). Because a 4-point decline is expected over 6 months (without therapy) in the average patient with AD, the rivastigmine–placebo difference of almost 5 points translates into a delay in progression of cognitive decline of potentially 6 months.

Further studies of the therapeutic effect of rivastigmine on cognition are being conducted in patients with severe AD, as well as those with vascular dementia.

Galantamine is a selective, reversible, competitive cholinesterase inhibitor that also allosterically modulates acetylcholine nicotinic receptors. The agent's modulatory effect on nicotinic receptors may potentiate the response of these receptors to acetylcholine. This enhancement of cholinergic nicotinic neurotransmission may be of clinical relevance because activation of presynaptic nicotinic receptors may stimulate the release of acetylcholine (Figure 19).

Galantamine has shown significant improvement in all measured domains of cognitive and global function (MMSE, ADAS-cog, CIBIC-plus). The clinical benefits for cognitive and ADL functions are maintained for at least 12 months. The compound is overall well tolerated, but cholinergic side-effects may occur. Patients receiving galantamine (16 and 24 mg/day) showed an improvement of 1–2 points above baseline in ADAS-cog scores; the magnitude of treatment effect with galantamine over placebo was documented, with 3–4 points on the ADAS-cog (Figure 20).

Long-term trials of galantamine versus placebo in patients with MCI have recently been started. Additional trials of galantamine in patients with presumed vascular dementia, as well as in individuals with presumed Lewy body dementia, are under way.

Summary: Based on results of various controlled clinical trials, all modern AChEIs produced statistically significant improvement of both cognitive and non-cognitive function (using standardized and validated rating scales/measures). There appears to be a similarity in magnitude of cognitive effect (compared to placebo), as well as a similarity in clinical effects. On average, almost one half of treated patients can be considered positive responders. Approximately 20% of patients

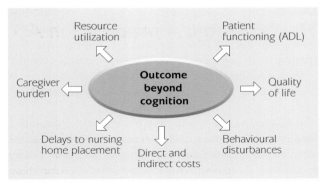

Figure 21. Outcomes beyond cognition in clinical trials.

do not improve on these AChEIs at a given dosage, the so-called non-responders.

There are unfortunately no characteristics that would help the clinician identify responders or non-responders before initiating the therapy.

Though the effects of therapy are similar, there may be differences between the agents that could translate into differences not only in the magnitude of the therapeutic effect, but in the duration of the clinical effect. Some of the outcome factors beyond cognition are depicted in Figure 21.

Evidence-based therapeutic recommendation

Several agents are currently available for the treatment of AD. To date, only some of these drugs have shown evidence of efficacy that would justify a recommendation for their therapeutic use. Based on the critical analysis of the literature (controlled clinical trials), only the approved AChEIs – donepezil, rivastigmine, galantamine (and tacrine) – are currently to be recommended under strict scientific criteria for use in the treatment of AD. Another valid option would be memantine (available in Europe).

The behavioural problems in AD

...Do not go gentle into that good night.
Rage, rage against the dying of the light.
Dylan Thomas

Behavioural disturbances and neuropsychiatric symptoms are common in AD (Table 16). They occur at some time during the course of the disease in nearly all patients. The behavioural problems most often cause severe distress to the caregiver, the family and to the patient himself. Behavioural and neuropsychiatric symptoms are strong predictors of institutionalization or nursing home placement. The caregiver can simply no longer handle the behaviourally disturbed patient alone. Managing behavioural symptoms therefore is of the highest priority for the clinician, since they may result in poorer functioning and are strong predictors of poorer prognosis.

The neuropsychiatric symptoms include psychosis, depression and anxiety. In the later stages of AD, the symptoms

Neuropsychiatric symptoms in AD	
Symptom	**% of Patients**
Apathy	50–70
Agitation	40–65
Anxiety	30–50
Irritability	30–45
Depression	40
Disinhibition	30–40
Delusions	20–40
Night behaviour	20–25
Hallucinations	5–15

Table 16. Neuropsychiatric symptoms in AD.

may include both agitation and physically aggressive behaviours, sundowning, disturbances of the diurnal rhythm, and insomnia. (Obstructive sleep apnoea may also develop at later stages.)

Psychosis

The term psychosis defines the clinical syndrome featuring delusions and hallucinations as principal symptoms. Delusions by definition are false beliefs based on incorrect inference about external reality and firmly held despite evidence to the contrary. Hallucinations by definition are sensory perceptions occurring without stimulation of the relevant sensory organ.

Delusions and hallucinations are common in AD patients; the most common delusions are those involving fear of theft, infidelity, abandonment and persecution (Table 17). Delusions can occur at any stage of the disease; they can even precede the memory decline. They are, however, most prominent in the middle, and especially the later stages of AD. Usually, patients with delusions show a more rapid deterioration in cognitive functions than those without. Patients with delusions present with a more disturbed behaviour than those without; they might be more aggressive, more anxious, more disrupted in their activity pattern. Delusions are one major reason for earlier institutionalization.

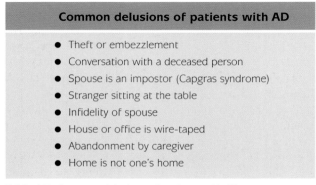

Common delusions of patients with AD

- Theft or embezzlement
- Conversation with a deceased person
- Spouse is an impostor (Capgras syndrome)
- Stranger sitting at the table
- Infidelity of spouse
- House or office is wire-taped
- Abandonment by caregiver
- Home is not one's home

Table 17. Common delusions of patients with AD.

Neuropathologically, patients with psychotic features show a higher amount of plaques and tangles in the medial temporal/prosubicular region and in the middle frontal cortex. The norepinephrine levels in the substantia nigra are also elevated, while the serotonin levels in the prosubiculum appear to be significantly lower. Though suggested, it is not yet established knowledge that the cholinergic deficit of AD contributes to the delusional disorder.

The frequency of hallucinations in AD patients (about 15–20%) is lower than that of delusions. One major reason for these false sensory impressions are sensory deficits in the elderly, that should be sought. The hallucinations can be auditory, visual or of another source. Some patients with AD experience visual hallucinations: seeing persons from the past, children playing in a house where there have formerly been children, possible intruders. These hallucinations frequently have their basis in past experiences of the individual. A patient with AD whose visual hallucinations were seeing horses running and himself chasing them had actually spent much of his life around horses.

Agitation

Agitation is a common finding in AD. It may occur in up to approximately 70% of all patients, and actually independently of other major behavioural disorders. It becomes more common as the disease advances. In our experience extreme agitation, especially in male AD patients, appear to be a last ditch effort to fight "the dying of the light". This agitated stage may then be followed by rapid physical deterioration into the final stages of AD. The phenomenon has multiple causes, and may be explained by the cholinergic deficit and frontal and temporal lobe dysfunction.

Agitation and aggression can be very distressing. This includes hitting, biting, tearing and pushing. They may be manifested by pacing, clapping, disrobing, making noises and then verbally aggressive behaviours including screaming, swearing, complaining and constantly asking for attention. Agitation is usually not well tolerated by the caregiver or in a nursing home setting. Therefore, these symptoms need to be urgently treated.

Anxiety

Many AD patients become very anxious. They may have agitated signs such as insomnia, loss of appetite and weight loss, which may be part of the anxiety syndrome or indicative of depression (Table 18). The symptoms of anxiety may mimic medical problems, with complaints of chest pain, palpitations and recurrent abdominal pain. There sometimes may be a real fixation about the symptoms. And then, in spite of frequent work-up and reassurance, there may be no resolution of some of these symptoms.

Depression

AD patients are more likely to express feelings of sadness and despair (Table 19). The final stages may be part of the picture of their giving up, refusing to eat, refusing to exercise or refusing to participate in any group activity. Depression can also severely disrupt the sleep pattern, with night and day reversal.

Sexual activity

There are several patterns of sexual expression to be seen in AD. While some patients present with mostly transient periods

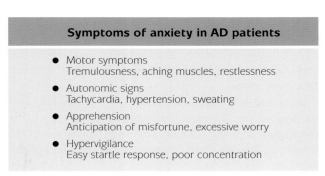

Symptoms of anxiety in AD patients

- Motor symptoms
  Tremulousness, aching muscles, restlessness
- Autonomic signs
  Tachycardia, hypertension, sweating
- Apprehension
  Anticipation of misfortune, excessive worry
- Hypervigilance
  Easy startle response, poor concentration

Table 18. Symptoms of anxiety in AD patients.

of attempted increased sexual activity or even inappropriate acting out of sexual aggressiveness, the majority of patients show diminished sexual interest.

Seizures

As many as 20–30% of all AD patients (usually late stage) have recurrent seizures or epilepsy during the course of their disease. Some seizures may follow recurrent cerebral vascular insults. One possible contributing cause to be considered is the toxicity of medication. Several drugs used in this population can lower the seizure threshold. Tricyclic antidepressants, antipsychotic drugs and cardiac antiarrhythmic drugs are among those predisposing to seizures.

Extrapyramidal signs

In addition to the frontal and parietal cholinergic deficit in AD, there is also a reduction in striatal dopamine. This may manifest itself with extrapyramidal signs such as bradykinesia, loss of facial expression, rigidity, and flexed posture. When these symptoms develop as an exaggerated response to a neuroleptic agent, the diagnosis of senile dementia of Lewy body type should be considered. When gait disorder precedes the

Symptoms of depression in AD patients
● Depressed mood most of the day
● Diminished pleasure in most activities
● Loss of appetite/weight loss
● Difficulty getting to sleep or staying asleep
● Psychomotor agitation/retardation
● Feelings of worthlessness/being a burden
● Impaired concentration/indecisiveness
● Recurring thoughts of death or suicide
● Diminished attention to grooming/hygiene

Table 19. Symptoms of depression in AD patients.

dementia, then other illnesses need to be looked for, especially vascular dementia. To some extent, the severity of extrapyramidal signs in patients with AD correlates with the severity of the dementia. Bradykinesia and hypomimia, for example, are present in up to 70% of patients with mild to moderate AD. The presence of extrapyramidal signs is associated with a more rapid progression and a worse prognosis.

Pharmacological treatment of behavioural and neuropsychiatric symptoms

The benzodiazepines may be most useful for the treatment of **anxiety** in AD. Shorter-acting agents such as lorazepam are preferred over the longer-acting agents. They are less likely to accumulate, and to produce weakness, ataxia or confusion. The risk of falls is then elevated. Some individuals will develop adverse reactions with hyperactivity. Also, buspiron may be an option for the treatment of anxiety in AD.

For the treatment of **depression** in AD, there is a recommendation from the American Psychiatric Association (1997) for use of selective serotonin reuptake inhibitors (SSRIs). These agents have a favourable side-effect profile, and have a lower risk for orthostatic hypotension than some of the tricyclic antidepressants, which additionally show anticholinergic properties. A list of drugs for the treatment of depression in AD patients is given in Table 20.

Effective agents for the management of **agitation** may be atypical antipsychotics, as well as anticonvulsants, antidepressants or anxiolytics (Table 21). Patients with hallucinations may respond well to haloperidol, which can, however, increase the cognitive impairment.

Insomnia and **sleep disturbances** can be treated with (short-acting) hypnotics, or trazodone. Drugs that cause strong sedation should generally be avoided, because of the risk of falls or other injuries.

Seizures in patients with AD respond well to anticonvulsant agents (Table 22). These medications may, however, not be well tolerated by all patients. Patients also need to be managed with strict attention to regular eating and sleeping patterns to minimize the number of seizures that could be attributable to malnutrition and metabolic changes or sleep deprivation.

Male patients exhibiting an inappropriate **sexual** drive may respond to hormonal treatment with medroxyprogesterone (300 mg/week, i.m.). Injections of leuprolide might also be successful in decreasing sexual aggression in males. Carbamazepine may

Drugs for the treatment of depression in AD	
Agent	**Dose range (mg/day)**
Sertraline	50–150
Paroxetine	10–30
Fluoxetine	5–30
Citalopram	20–40
Venlafaxine	50–300
Trazodone	50–200
Desipramine	50–100

Table 20. Drugs for the treatment of depression in AD.

Drugs for the treatment of agitation in AD	
Agent	**Dose range (mg/day)**
Risperidone	0.5–1.5
Olanzapine	5–10
Quetiapine	25–100
Haloperidol	0.5–3
Trazodone	50–300
Carbamazepine	200–1000
Valproate	250–1000
Buspirone	15–45
Lorazepam	0.5–6

Table 21. Drugs for the treatment of agitation in AD.

be of benefit in patients with sexual disturbances as part of Kluver–Bucy syndrome, a complex behavioural disorder consisting of hyperorality, hypermetamorphosis, emotional placidity, agnosia and altered sexual behaviour. It may occur in fragmentary form (with masturbation, apathy, agnosia, mouthing behaviour) in late stages of AD.

There is some evidence from more recent studies that AChEIs might have favourable effects on behavioural symptoms in patients with AD. The available agents (donepezil, rivastigmine, galantamine) have all been shown to reduce behavioural disturbances in patients with AD, with significant effects on apathy, anxiety, disinhibition and depression/dysphoria.

Delusions and **hallucinations** in patients with AD can be treated with conventional neuroleptic agents. There is, however, the rather high risk of developing extrapyramidal dysfunction and further cognitive impairment as characteristic side-effects. The recently introduced so-called atypical antipsychotics might therefore be the better choice. These agents have a complex receptor activity profile and are reported to exert their antipsychotic efficacy through effects on non-D_2 receptors, which makes them less likely to produce extrapyramidal side-effects. The conventional antipsychotics are known to be primarily active at the D_2 dopamine receptor. The commonly used antipsychotics are listed in Table 23.

Antiepileptic drugs for the treatment of seizures in AD patients	
Agent	**Dose range (mg/day)**
Phenytoin	300–400
Carbamazepine	400–1000
Divalproex	750–1500

Table 22. Antiepileptic drugs for the treatment of seizures in AD patients.

Generally, the pharmacological approach in patients with dementia should be very careful – start low, go slow – based on experience and following the established treatment guidelines (Table 24).

Non-pharmacological approach

Providing meaningful activities, appropriate stimulation, loving care and being aware of precipitants as well as a calming environment can help a lot in either avoiding behavioural disturbances or managing neuropsychiatric symptoms. Recreational activities can combat depression, sadness and loneliness; exercise during the day improves sleep quality.

Good nutrition/patiently feeding and providing appetite-stimulating food can lift the mood and stimulate the patient for (other) pleasant activities. Loving and understanding care helps to cope with disinhibition and sexual aggression.

The noise level, the lighting and the furnishing of the place where the patient lives influences the risk of hallucinations and delusions. A secure environment provides room for mobility but keeps the patients from running away.

As agitation and aggression can be caused by painful medical or orthopaedic conditions, which the patient can no longer articulate, further medical/orthopaedic work-up is to be considered. If aggressive behaviour occurs during special

Antipsychotics for the treatment of delusions and hallucinations in AD	
Agent	**Dose range (mg/day)**
Risperidone	0.5–1.5
Olanzapine	5–10
Quetiapine	25–100
Thioridazine	30–150
Haloperidol	0.5–3

Table 23. Antipsychotics for the treatment of delusions and hallucinations in AD.

occasions, for example when being dressed or while toileting, then the provoking reason may be actual physical pain.

Some practical ways for caregivers to reduce and to manage frequently occurring behavioural problems are listed in Table 25.

Guidelines for the pharmacotherapy of behaviour disturbances in dementia

Before prescribing

Establish accurate diagnosis, document concurrent illness and monitor comorbidities.

Take careful medication history (including OTC drugs).

Limit use of medications and look for non-pharmacological alternatives where possible.

Do not avoid pharmacotherapy just because of age or "anyway bad prognosis".

When prescribing

Choose specific target symptoms for pharmacological treatment and carefully monitor the response.

Provide simple written instructions for patient and caregiver.

Use low doses initially, but do not hesitate to increase doses in small steps if necessary for a sufficient effect (obtain serum drug levels as help for dosage decisions).

Choose drugs for concurrent diseases that do not cause deterioration of cognition and functional ability.

Know the potential side-effects and the potential interactions.

Avoid multiple drug regimes.

After prescribing

Evaluate compliance and response.

Accept partial response if better effects would mean unacceptable side-effects.

Review drug regime regularly and discontinue unnecessary medications.

Ask regularly about side-effects and monitor adverse events.

Source: adapted from Cummings, J.L. (1999) Education Program Syllabus. Am. Acad. Neurol.

Table 24. Guidelines for the pharmacotherapy of behaviour disturbances in dementia.

How to deal with behavioural problems typical for AD

Behaviour	What to do
Indecision	Reduce choices
Poor memory	Provide notepads, calendars, portraits of children/grandchildren with names on
Sundowning	Exercise earlier in the day, keep evening environment calm, well lit
Apathy	Initiate activities that patient can complete
Relocation stress	Move during daylight, keep memorabilia from home accessible
Wandering	Exercise, provide safe place for mobility, keep ID on patient
Not eating	Reduce distractions at meal times, offer easy-to-eat finger food, offer in-between snacks, provide nicely prepared food (feast for eyes)
Bored, restless	Provide music, old videos, family photos, picture books

Table 25. How to deal with behavioural problems typical for AD.

Guidelines for the diagnosis of dementia

During the last 15 years there have been several guidelines or consensus statements published by various organizations and states. Unfortunately, they differ considerably in several aspects, therefore offering diverse recommendations to the clinician for the diagnostic process. Some also include recommendations for treatment.

Some published guidelines reflect expert opinions, while others are based on the advice of an advisory panel, including a peer review process. Some, however, can be considered evidence based (Table 26).

By giving different recommendations for procedures and office-based work-up, using these guidelines generates costs of variable amount. The higher costs of diagnosis in some of the guidelines are mainly driven by imaging techniques, such as PET. Interestingly and conversely, most guidelines do not recommend neuroimaging as part of the routine assessment, thus carrying the risk of overlooking many severe diseases that could cause dementia.

Another criterion, with marked differences in recommendation, addresses the referral to specialists (neurologist, psychiatrist, neuropsychologist, geriatrician) for differential diagnosis. It should, however, be widely accepted by now that a disease such as AD requires a multidisciplinary team approach.

Evidence-based guidelines for the diagnosis of dementia

- American Academy of Neurology (1994)
- US Agency for Health Care Policy and Research (1996)
- Canadian Consensus Conference on Dementia (1999)

Table 26. Evidence-based guidelines for the diagnosis of dementia.

Guidance on the use of AChEIs

In view of the fact that new therapies are emerging and becoming available for the first time for the treatment of patients with AD, regarding which only limited experience has yet been gained, the UK-based National Institute for Clinical Excellence (NICE) has recently published a "Guidance on the Use of Donepezil, Rivastigmine, and Galantamine for the Treatment of Alzheimer's Disease" (NICE, 2001). This guidance represents the view of the institute's appraisal committee. The document has been reviewed by a number of groups, governmental and non-governmental organizations, and various institutions, and is supposed to reflect current knowledge and medical practice.

The main demand of the paper is the following: the three new AChEIs – donepezil, rivastigmine and galantamine – should be made available in the National Health Service (NHS) (under defined conditions) as one component of the management of those people with mild and moderate AD, whose MMSE score is above 12 points.

Prognostic factors in AD

A prognostic judgement concerning the individual patient with AD is still not possible. There are, however, several features that are either positively associated or inversely correlated with progression and deterioration, as well as with prolonged survival. Factors of good prognosis include mild dementia, independence in ADL and lack of depression. Factors of bad prognosis include young age at onset, early institutionalization, psychotic symptoms and the development of extrapyramidal signs (EPSs).

The general survival of a patient with clinically overt AD is, on average, 10.3 years (with a broad range from a few months to 21 years). Patients with AD show a longer survival time than those with vascular or the mixed form of AD and vascular dementia. An earlier age of onset of symptoms was, in some studies, correlated with a more rapid progression and shorter survival time (a controversial finding).

ApoE4 allele carriers show a higher mortality but a slower cognitive decline. The cognitive decline is also slower in patients with a high educational level.

Among the clinical features, the initial severity of the dementia is related to the survival. The (negative) prognostic value of aphasia remains controversial. Severe impairments of visuospatial function and immediate recall have been identified as worsening the prognosis.

Aggressive acting out behaviour is recognized as a feature that seems to predict a faster decline. Falls, especially those causing hip fractures, seem to increase the likelihood of death. Neuropsychiatric symptoms such as hallucinations or paranoia may also be associated with a more rapid progression of the disease.

Among the most robust negative prognostic factors, resulting in rapid or faster decline, are frontal lobe dysfunctions and EPSs. EPSs have also been linked to increased mortality in AD.

Comprehensive and loving care

*…Darling, do you remember
the man you married? Touch me,
remind me who I am.*
Stanley Kunitz

It is surprising to observe what difference care can make for the patient with AD, who in the later stages can no longer articulate his wishes, feelings or needs, and who has unlearned how to eat, how to use silver, how to swallow, how to dress, how to toilet. Regular, patient feeding, for example with food that stimulates the appetite by smell and appearance – even if eaten with the fingers – protects the patient from gradual starvation and loss of weight. Malnutrition is definitely not part of the ordinary disease process, but rather a sad sign of neglect.

One sensation, however, remains for a long period spared by the devastating disease: even in extremely apathetic or delusioned patients the emotional sensitivity is present. Loving care and attention therefore should never be abolished or exchanged for qualified routine care. AD patients – like newborn babies – enjoy deeply every form of skin contact; stroking usually helps in calming the patients down. It gives comfort and security and makes the patient feel better.

Better treatment of pain

Pain appears to be frequently undertreated in cognitively impaired older adults, particularly in nursing home residents. One reason for this is the reduced language skill associated with difficulties in finding words and in articulation. One rather obvious sign of pain may be increased irritability or aggressive behaviour. Also, changes in sleep pattern, loss of appetite and resistance to personal care are possible signs of untreated or undertreated pain in AD patients.

As instruments to detect pain in non-verbal, cognitively impaired patients are still in the developmental stages, there are other observational hints instead to be utilized, which may signify pain. Crying out, for example, might be a form of vocalizing pain. Facial expressions such as forehead wrinkling, wincing and grimacing may be used by the patient to show pain. Increased restlessness, grabbing on to furniture, moving extremely slowly, difficulty lying down or getting up – all may be a sign of pain, which otherwise can no longer be expressed.

How to communicate with the patient

As the AD patient loses his cognitive and language skills, communication becomes difficult. The patient, on the one hand, might no longer be able to articulate his needs. The caregiver, on the other hand, needs to use simple words and communication strategies for the management of the patient. Misunderstandings and conflicts are frequent, but can often be avoided. Table 27 lists a series of tips for an effective communication with the deteriorating AD patient.

Tips for effective communication with the patient

- Touch and establish eye contact.
- Beckon; use gestures to augment words; hold hands out; be friendly; smile.
- Be attentive to messages communicated by the patient's body position and movement.
- Find a quiet setting; reduce environmental confusion.
- Speak in concise, clear and short sentences.
- Construct sentences using words the patient uses.
- Take advantage of calm moments to express warmth and caring with a gentle touch.
- Aberrant behaviour is less likely to be motivated by unconscious conflicts than by needs or fears.
- Listen to the patient even though the words may not make sense.
- Keep voice calm, low and reasonably modulated.
- If unable to attract the patient's attention, leave and try again some minutes later.
- The patient may respond to verbalization very slowly; don't rush and allow sufficient time.

Table 27. Tips for effective communication with the patient.

How the patient communicates with you

Patients with severe AD may communicate emotions and needs by squeezing a caregiver's arm, facial and body language or even moans. Some may find a last vehicle for expressing their emotions by taking up previously learned musical skills, dancing or painting. The picture, shown in Figure 22, was painted by a woman with AD who could no longer speak. She would pat her chest and gesture as if trying to release feelings from her heart.

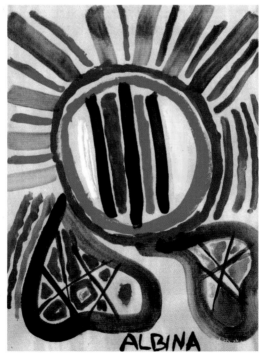

Figure 22. Title of water colour by Albina: "My Radiant Heart". Courtesy of Charles and Marjean Cole, representing the "Drawing on Memories" program of the Oklahoma Alzheimer's Association.

Caring for the caregiver

Once the diagnosis of AD is determined, the physician has to deal with two patients: the demented person and the caregiver. Given the progressive course of the disease, the immense burden the caregiver has to carry should be taken into account. Not only is the caregiver (if part of the family or the spouse) all of a sudden losing a beloved person and/or partner, but a deep shadow also falls on their personal future. Seeing someone you love suffer from AD is a major stress; caring for that particular person is even more stressful. Providing as much support as possible for the major caregiver is therefore one of the important tasks of the physician who deals with Alzheimer's patients.

As soon as a diagnosis of AD is suspected, the physician and other health care providers need to inform and advise the patient's family, and especially the direct caregiver, concerning the expected progressive course of the disease. The responsible caregiver might need further help initially to learn how to cope with the emerging situation. Too often the caring person is neglected, which can result in a severe depression or other illness, not to mention the social isolation over the years the care of an Alzheimer's patient is associated with. There is also a need for psychological support and advice, as many caregivers feel guilty when they cannot perform optimal care or have to place the patient in a nursing home or other facility.

In many cases, it is not the care taking per se that brings the heaviest burden, but the behavioural problems the patient with AD might develop. Some of them can and should be treated vigorously, but some of them cannot be treated pharmacologically.

It is the behavioural problems that in most cases finally give reason for the institutionalization of a patient. Restlessly wandering, running away, aggression, delusions, sleep disturbance and sundowning, or eating problems are frequently occurring features. In these cases it certainly is of advantage for the patient as well as for the caregiver to find a safe place and a facility, where the patient can be managed and good care can be provided around the clock.

There is also a very practical aspect for integrating the caregiver into the therapeutic team: he or she has to provide the treatment and provide the information for further evaluations during the follow-up.

The physician can take part in providing social support (particularly concerning home services, support groups, day care, nursing home placement, etc.) and can deliver information about necessary legal and financial matters that have to be handled. In AD, it is of importance to make careful plans in advance.

Possible future approaches

Apolipoprotein E genotyping

Apolipoprotein E (ApoE) is a naturally formed protein that helps carry blood cholesterol throughout the body. ApoE occurs with three different alleles: ApoE2, ApoE3 and ApoE4. Each person has a gene that codes for one of these versions. Since genes are present in pairs, there exist six possible combinations. Research has shown that, when individuals carry the ApoE4 allele, they are particularly at risk for the development of sporadic and late-onset familial AD, whereas the ApoE2 allele seems to be protective. Thus, genotyping could possibly help to identify persons at risk for AD and make it possible to introduce either preventive or early treatments.

In addition to its role in the lipid transport system, ApoE performs multiple other metabolic tasks. ApoE interacts with many proteins, including beta-peptide. Future drug development for prevention or early treatment of AD includes the identification of the specific molecular interactions of ApoE.

Cholinergic activity enhancers and muscarinic agonists

Selective muscarinic (M1) agonists may still be effective after loss of presynaptic cholinergic neurons. Evidence suggests that the postsynaptic muscarinic receptor system remains relatively intact, even in moderately affected patients.

Beta-amyloid is known to be deposited in the brains of AD patients. The amyloid plaques formed are believed to be the primary cause of the neurodegeneration in AD. If a muscarinic agonist proves effective in reducing the concentrations of beta-amyloid in the brain, this could be an important step towards prevention.

Researchers hope that muscarinic agonists that stimulate M_1 or M_3 receptors will yet prove an effective therapy for AD.

Thus far, clinical efficacy has not been demonstrated in initial trials with M_1 agonists in AD. Newer muscarinic agonists, possibly used in combination with AChEIs or other agents, may show better results.

Nicotinic agents

Nicotinic agents presumably work presynaptically at autoreceptors to raise levels of acetylcholine within the synapse. Galantamine is the first approved drug which modulates the nicotinic receptor. Other agents are in development.

Nicotinic receptors play a role in learning and memory. Two nicotinic acetylcholine receptors (nAChRs) are identified and characterized: a 7 subtype, which mediates a rapidly decaying current, and a 42 subtype, which mediates a slowly decaying current. The number of nAChRs in the frontal and temporal cortices appears to be reduced in the brains of AD patients.

Antioxidants

Findings in recent studies support the hypothesis that systemic oxidative stress is associated with cognitive decline, or, in other words, that increased levels of oxidative stress and/or antioxidant deficiencies, as well as poor antioxidant status, may pose risk factors for cognitive impairment. These findings could encourage the evaluation or development of antioxidants as a preventative or therapeutic strategy against cognitive decline and with this against possible AD in the elderly.

Combination therapy using statins, oestrogen and anti-inflammatory agents

This has not yet been studied in detail, but certainly a feasible option would be the combination therapy of AChEIs with either oestrogens, antioxidants, statins or anti-inflammatory agents. One recent trial combining an AChEI with a cyclo-oxygenase-2 (COX-2) inhibitor, however, did not show clinical efficacy.

Other agents in development

AIT-082 (Neotrofin) is a hypoxanthine derivative which passes the blood–brain barrier and appears to mimic the effects of neurotrophic factors. Studies in patients with mild to moderate AD are now underway to assess efficacy and safety.

FK960 is an aminopiperazine, whose efficacy appears to result from its effect on synaptic plasticity. The compound enhances the release of somatostatin from the hippocampus. FK960 does not bind to cholinergic receptors nor does it inhibit AChE. Studies are now being conducted in patients with mild to moderate AD.

DVD742 is a selective GABA-B antagonist, which demonstrates efficacy in memory and learning in a variety of animal models. Its psychopharmacologic features suggest that it may improve memory and cognition in humans, and is now being tested in patients with mild cognitive impairment (MCI).

Other approaches in preclinical development include: anti-NFT agents to decrease the production of NFTs in neurons to prevent neuronal dysfunction and cell death, and anti-apoptotic agents, to stop the programmed neuronal death.

Protease inhibitors – prevention of beta-amyloid formation

Alpha-, beta- and gamma-secretases play a role in the fragmentation of amyloid precursor protein (APP), from which the toxic beta-amyloid (as a small fragment) is derived. Beta-amyloid in AD patients is cut off the full-length APP molecule by beta- and gamma-secretases at a "wrong" site. This results in the deposition of beta-amyloid in amyloid plaques, which are considered as major contributors to the pathology in AD. Gamma-secretase seems to be closely associated with presenilin 1, a membrane protein, which when mutated causes autosomal dominant AD. These rather new findings make beta- and gamma-secretases logical candidates for specific therapeutic inhibition. They are currently under development by major pharmaceutical companies.

Beta-amyloid immunization

The classic neuritic plaque is characterized by a central core of beta-amyloid. Surrounding this core is a nest of inflammation and injury, where activated microglial cells, astroglia and proteases can be found.

Immunizing the patient with AD against beta-amyloid with antibodies targeted to beta-amyloid is another potential treatment strategy. This has proven successful in transgenic mice that overproduce beta-amyloid (Figure 23). Such immunization resulted in no further accumulation (and even some degree of regression) of neuritic plaques in these mice brains. These findings raise the possibility of immunization that might prevent and reverse the pathological cascade. Initial AN1792 vaccine trials in patients with AD are underway.

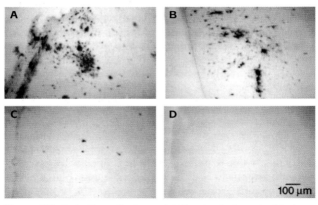

Figure 23. Reduction of beta-amyloid burden in the entorhinal and retrosplenial cortex of older PDAPP transgenic mice following beta-amyloid injection. Beta-amyloid deposition in the retrosplenial (RSC) and entorhinal (EC) cortices of 15-month-old PBS- (**A**,**B**) and beta-amyloid 42-injected mice (**C**,**D**). Beta-amyloid deposition was greatly reduced in the RSC of beta-amyloid-injected mice compared with the PBS group (compare **A** and **C**). No beta-amyloid was detected in the EC of beta-amyloid 42-injected mice (**D**), in contrast to the PBS group (**B**). Reproduced with permission from Schenk, D (1999) Immunization with amyloid-beta attenuates Alzheimer-disease-like pathology in the PDAPP mouse. *Nature* **400,** 173–177. Copyright © 1999 Macmillan Magazines Ltd.

Stem cell therapy

The use of embryonic stem cells for the renewal of damaged tissues and restoration of impaired functions is probably one of the most exciting developments for the future. In no area of medicine is the potential of stem cell research greater than in diseases of the nervous system. In AD, for example, cells that release acetylcholine die. Supplying new cells to the vulnerable structures of the brain is an intriguing thought. Experimental cell replacement therapies are already under way.

A group of researchers at the University of Illinois, for example, injected neural stem cells from aborted human foetuses into 24-month-old rats (equivalent in age to people about 80 years old). The cells developed into neurons and other brain cells. When tested for their ability to learn and remember, the rats scored better than they had before getting the transplants, on average doing as well as young adult rats.

Human pluripotent stem cells could be grown in culture and then transplanted to brain areas either as pluripotent stem cells or after being treated to become a specific type of neural cell. Work in animal models of human nervous system diseases has provided evidence that mouse pluripotent stem cells can survive, differentiate and give some degree of functional recovery following transplantation to the affected region of the nervous system. In addition, stem cells could be stimulated to eventually develop into a cell type that uses dopamine to transmit signals between nerve cells (of particular interest for Parkinson's disease). Similar approaches could be developed to replace the dead or dysfunctional cells in cortical and hippocampal brain regions affected in patients with AD.

Additionally, stem cells could be used as vectors for delivering genes or other therapeutic substances, such as neurotrophic or growth factors, to defined brain regions. Human pluripotent stem cells thus offer the potential to deliver therapeutic molecules to brain regions that are undergoing cell atrophy, as seen in ageing or cell death in AD.

Concluding remarks

Until recently, there was no symptomatic therapy available for the treatment of the primary deficits of progressive memory loss and cognitive decline in patients with AD. Now, new therapies have been tested and released to the public which are having a modest but significant impact upon the ravages of the disease. Numerous promising therapeutic interventions have entered testing phases. There is now hope for significant breakthroughs in AD treatment, as well as for a more satisfying routine management, as pointed out by Dennis J. Selkoe, Boston, in an editorial in the *JAMA* (2000, Vol. 283, No 12):

"In the future, it is likely that individuals entering their fifth or sixth decade of life will undergo a formal AD risk assessment as part of routine health maintenance. This assessment most likely will include a careful exploration of family history for AD or other dementias, a blood screen for relevant gene defects underlying AD, measurement of plasma Abeta levels and, when indicated, determination of cerebrospinal fluid levels of Abeta42, tau, and other markers of the neuropathology. Based on quantitative algorithms of risk, individuals could be offered preventive treatment. […] If even partial success is achieved, society will need to grapple with the eventuality that many more people may survive into late age with little or no cognitive impairment, a welcome problem indeed."

Resources

Useful addresses and internet links

Alzheimer's Association
For caregivers: offers a wealth of information, particularly for
the caregiver, on patient and symptom management, legal
issues, etc. Handouts (practical and educational) are
available in national editions and various languages.
Hotline: (800) 272-3900 www.alz.org
http://www.alzheimers.com
For physicians: the Association maintains a separate section on
its website specifically for physicians and other health care
professionals. This site offers information on diagnosis,
treatment and clinical trials, as well as useful links to
additional resources within and outside the Association.
www.alz.org/hc

Alzheimer's Disease Association
Hotline: (212) 983-0700

Alzheimer's Disease Education & Referral Center
The ADEAR Center is a service of the National Institute of
Aging. Visitors will find information about Alzheimer's
disease and related dementias (news, publications,
research). Links to other federal resources.
P.O. Box 8250, Silver Spring, MD 20907-8250
Email: adear@alzheimers.org www.alzheimers.org
Hotline: (800) 438-4380

Alzheimer Disease Research Center,
Washington University
www.adrc.wustl.edu

American Association of Retired Persons (AARP)

Free information on Alzheimer's disease and resources in
the community. Caregiver resource kit can be provided.

601 E. Street, NW, Washington, DC 20049
Email: member@aarp.org **www.aarp.org**

Alzheimer Europe

www.alzheimer-europe.org

Dementia Web

www.dementia.ion.ucl.ac.uk

Institute on Aging (University of Pennsylvania)

Offers links to ageing-related research, education and
clinical care. Educational programmes and publications.

University of Pennsylvania, 3615 Chestnut Street
Philadelphia, PA 19104-6006
Phone: (215) 898-3163
Email: ageweb@mail.med.upenn.edu
www.med.upenn.edu/aging

National Institutes of Health

Broad spectrum of information, publications, library
services, databases, trial information.

Public Information Office, Building 31, Room 2B10
9000 Rockville Pike, Bethesda, MD 20892
Phone: (301) 496-1766
National Institute on Aging: (301) 496-1752.
www.ninds.nih.gov/health_and_medical/disorders/
alzheimersdisease_doc.htm

American Geriatrics Society

Works to promote effective, high-quality research that addresses health care problems of older people and expands knowledge of the ageing process. Offers physician and patient services.

Empire State Building, 350 Fifth Avenue, Suite 801, New York, NY 10118

Phone: (212) 308-1414

Email: info.amger@americangeriatrics.org

www.americangeriatrics.org

American Geriatrics Society Foundation for Health in Aging (FHA)

Building the bridge between research and practice of geriatric health care professionals and the public; advocates on behalf of older adults and their special needs. Offers physician and patient services.

Empire State Building, 350 Fifth Avenue, Suite 801, New York, NY 10118

Phone: (212) 755-6810

Email: staff@healthinaging.org www.healthinaging.org

American Association for Geriatric Psychiatry

7910 Woodmont Avenue, Suite 1050 Bethesda, MD 20814

Phone: (301) 654-7850 **Email:** main@aagpgpa.org

www.aagpgpa.org

American Academy of Neurology

1080 Montreal Avenue, St. Paul, MN 55116

Phone: (651) 695-1940 **Email:** web@aan.com

www.aan.com

Benjamin B. Green-Field National Alzheimer's Library and Resource Center

The Center houses an extensive collection of books and periodicals on AD and related disorders. Online access to its catalogue, selected reading lists. Health care professionals can request interlibrary loans and other reference assistance by calling **(312) 335-9602**. www.alz.org/aboutus/library

WebMD

A reference for the latest health and wellness information; publishes news articles and reference materials on diverse topics. Information is presented clearly enough for non-physicians to understand. **www.webmd.com**

Elder Web

Designed for caregivers, family, health care professionals, professional advisors of elderly people with needs. **www.elderweb.com**

Elderconnect

Extended care and home care information network providing extended care assistance, news and advice. Information on 35,000 providers nationwide in the USA, including community services and resources, assisted living apartments, and retirement units. **www.elderconnect.com**

Alzheimer's Disease Society

Gordon House
10 Greencoat Place
London SW1P 1PH

Alzheimer's Disease International

45/46 Lower Marsh
London SE1 7RG

Age Concern England

Astral House
1268 London Road
London SW16

Suggested reading and references

Books

Gauthier, S. (ed.) (1999) *Clinical Diagnosis and Management of Alzheimer's Disease*, 2nd edition. Martin Dunitz.

Geldmacher, D.S. (2001) *Contemporary Diagnosis and Management of Alzheimer's Disease*. Newtown, PA: Handbooks in Health Care.

Growdon, J.H.; Rossor, M.N. (eds) (1998) *The Dementias. Blue Books of Practical Neurology*. Butterworth-Heinemann.

Iqbal, K.; Swaab, D.F.; Winblad, B.; Wisniewski, H.M. (eds) (1999) *Alzheimer's Disease and Related Disorders. Etiology, Pathogenesis and Therapeutics*. John Wiley.

Mittelman, M.S. *et al.* (2000) *Guiding the Alzheimer's Caregiver. A Handbook for Counselors*. New York University School of Medicine.

Morris, J.C. (ed.) (1994) *Handbook of Dementing Illnesses*. Marcel Dekker.

National Institute for Clinical Excellence (NICE) (2001) Guidance on the use of donepezil, rivastigmine and galantamine for the treatment of Alzheimer's disease. *Technology Appraisal Guidance* No. 19 (January). London: NICE.

Pulst, S.-M. (ed.) (2000) *Neurogenetics*. Oxford University Press.

Quan, M. (ed.) (2001) *Clinical Cornerstone – Dementia. Excerpta Medica*, Volume 3, Number 4.

Richter, R.W.; Blass, J.P. (1994) *Alzheimer's Disease – A Guide to Practical Management*. Mosby.

Scinto, L.F.M.; Daffner, K.R. (eds) (2000) *Early Diagnosis of Alzheimer's Disease*. Humana Press.

World Health Organization (1999) Project on the development of methodologies for the early diagnosis, prevention, and treatment of Alzheimer's disease. http://www.who.int/msa/mnh/nrs/neuro1.htm. Accessed November 1999.

Articles

American Academy of Neurology (1994) Practice parameter for diagnosis and evaluation of dementia (summary statement). Report of the Quality Standards Subcommittee of the American Academy of Neurology. *Neurology* **44,** 2203–2206.

American Psychiatric Association (1997) Practice guidelines for the treatment of patients with Alzheimer's disease and other dementias of late life. *Am. J. Psychiat.* **154** (suppl. 5), 1–39.

Berr, C. *et al.* (2000) Cognitive decline is associated with systemic oxidative stress: the EVA study. *J. Am. Geriatr. Soc.* **48,** 1285–1291.

Blass, J.P.; Gibson, G.E. (1991) The role of oxidative abnormalities in the pathophysiology of Alzheimer's disease. *Rev. Neurol. (Paris)* **147,** 513–525.

Broe, G.A. *et al.* (2000) Anti-inflammatory drugs protect against Alzheimer's disease at low doses. *Arch. Neurol.* **57** (11), 1586–1591.

Corey-Bloom, J. *et al.* (1998) A randomized trial evaluating the efficacy and safety of ENA 713 (rivastigmine tartrate), a new acetylcholinesterase inhibitor, in patients with mild to moderately severe Alzheimer's disease. *Int. J. Geriatr. Psychopharmacol.* **1,** 55–65.

Costa, P.T. Jr *et al.* (1996) Recognition and initial assessment of Alzheimer's disease and related dementias. *Clinical Practice Guideline* No. 19. Rockville, MD: Department of Health and Human Services (US), Public Health Service, Agency for Health Care Policy and Research; AHCPR Publication No. 97-0702.

Doody, R.S. *et al.* (2001) Practice parameter: management of dementia (an evidence-based review). *Neurology* **56,** 1154–1166.

Dubinsky, R.M. *et al.* (2000) Practice parameter: risk of driving and Alzheimer's disease (an evidence-based review). *Neurology* **54,** 2205–2211.

Ernst, R.L.; Hay, J.W. (1994) The US economic and social costs of Alzheimer's disease revisited. *Am. J. Public Health* **84** (8), 1261–1264.

FDA (1989) Peripheral and Central Nervous System Drugs Advisory Committee (7 July). Rockville MD: Department of Health and Human Services, Public Health Service, Food and Drug Administration, pp. 213–214.

FDC Reports, Inc. (1992) FDA guidance on Alzheimer's drug clinical utility assessments. *FDC Reports* (*The Pink Sheet*) **54** (2 March), 13–15.

Feldman, H. *et al.* (2001) A 24-week randomized, double-blind study of donepezil in moderate to severe Alzheimer's disease. *Neurology* **57,** 613–620.

Giacobini, E. (2000) Cholinesterase inhibitors stabilize Alzheimer's disease. *Ann. N.Y. Acad. Sci.* **920,** 321–327.

Hachinski, V.; Munoz, D.G. (1997) Cerebrovascular pathology in Alzheimer's disease: cause effect or epiphenomenon? *Ann. N.Y. Acad. Sci.* **826,** 1–6.

Harrington, M.G. *et al.* (1986) Abnormal proteins in the cerebrospinal fluid of patients with Creutzfeldt–Jakob disease. *N. Engl. J. Med.* **315,** 279–283.

Knopman, D.S. *et al.* (2000) Patterns of care in the early stages of Alzheimer's disease: impediments to timely diagnosis. *J. Am. Geriatr. Soc.* **48,** 300–304.

Knopman, D.S. *et al.* (2001) Practice parameter: diagnosis of dementia (an evidence-based review). *Neurology* **56,** 1143–1153.

Larson, E.B. (1998) Management of Alzheimer's disease in a primary care setting. *Am. J. Geriatr. Psychiat.* **6** (suppl. 1), S34–S40.

Markesbery, W.R.; Ehmann, W.D. (1993) Aluminium and Alzheimer's disease. *Clin. Neurosci.* **1,** 212–218.

McKhann, G. *et al.* (1984) Clinical diagnosis of Alzheimer's disease: Report of the NINCDS-ADRDA Work Group under the auspices of Department of Health and Human Services Task Force on Alzheimer's Disease. *Neurology* **34,** 939–944.

Mohs, R.C. *et al.* (1983) Neuropathologically validated scales for Alzheimer's disease. In: Crook, T.; Ferris, S.; Bartus, R. (eds), *Assessment in Geriatric Psychopharmacology*. New Canaan, CT: Mark Powley.

Mohs, R.C. *et al.* (2001) A 1-year, placebo-controlled preservation of function survival study of donepezil in AD patients. *Neurology* **57,** 481–488.

Mondadori, C.; Jaeckel, J.; Preiswerk G. (1993) The first orally active GABA-B blocker improves the cognitive performance of mice, rats, and Rhesus monkeys. *Behav. Neurol. Biol.* **60,** 62–68.

Patterson, C.J.S. *et al.* (1999) The recognition, assessment and management of dementing disorders: conclusions from the Canadian Consensus Conference on Dementia. *Can. Med. Assoc. J.* **160** (suppl. 12), S1–S15.

Petersen, R.C. *et al.* (2001) Practice parameter: early detection of dementia: mild cognitive impairment (an evidence-based review). *Neurology* **56,** 1133–1142.

Reisberg, B.; Ferris, S.H. *et al.* (1988) Global deterioration scale (GDS). *Psychopharmacol. Bull.* **24,** 661–663.

Richter, R.W.; Farlow, M.R. (1998) Recent advances in the treatment of Alzheimer's disease. *J. Oklahoma State Med. Assoc.* **91** (8), 431-437.

Richter, R.W. *et al.* (1998) Neurotoxic syndromes. In: Rosenberg R.N.; Pleasure D.E. (eds), *Comprehensive Neurology*, 2nd edition, 851–887. Chichester: Wiley and Sons.

Rogers, S.L. *et al.* (1998) A 24-weeks, double-blind, placebo-controlled trial of donepezil in patients with Alzheimer's disease. *Neurology* **50,** 136–145.

Ronald and Nancy Reagan Research Institute of the Alzheimer's Association and the National Institute on Aging Working Group (1998) Consensus Report of the Working Group on Molecular and Biochemical Markers of Alzheimer's Disease. *Neurobiol. Aging* **19,** 109–116.

Rosenberg, R.N.; Richter R.W. *et al*. (1996) Genetic factors for the development of Alzheimer disease in the Cherokee Indian. *Arch. Neurol*. **53**, 997–1000.

Schenk, D. *et al*. (1999) Immunization with amyloid-beta attenuates Alzheimer-disease-like pathology in the PDAPP mouse. *Nature* **400** (8 July), 173–177.

Selkoe, D.J. (2000) The origins of Alzheimer disease. Editorial. *JAMA* **283** (12), 1615–1617.

Silverman, D.H. *et al*. (2001) Positron emission tomography in evaluation of dementia. *JAMA* **286,** 2120–2127.

Tariot, P.N. *et al*. (2000) A 5-month, randomized, placebo-controlled trial of galantamine in AD. *Neurology* **54**, 2269–2276.

Winblad B *et al*. (2001) A 1-year randomized, placebo controlled study of donepezil in patients with mild to moderate AD. *Neurology* **57,** 489–495.

Winblad, B.; Poritis, N.; Moebius, H.J. (1999) Clinical improvement in a placebo-controlled trial with memantine in care-dependent patients with severe dementia. In: Iqbal, K. *et al*. (eds), *Alzheimer's Disease,* 633–640. Chichester: Wiley and Sons.

Veld BA *et al*. (2001) ANon-steroidalantiinflammatory drugs and the risk of Alzheimer's disease. *N. Engl. J. Med*. **345,** 1515–1521.

Zoeller, B. *et al*. (2001) Rational therapy of Alzheimer's disease based on the outcome and significance of recent clinical trials. *Schweiz. Rundsch. Med. Praxis* **90,** 827–834.

Appendix

The UK National Service Framework for Older People

The UK government produces occasional National Service Frameworks (NSFs) – standards of treatment and healthcare for the UK.

The "NSF for Older People" contains seven standards. The one of most relevance to Alzheimer's disease (AD) is Standard 7, that: *"Older people who have mental health problems have access to integrated mental health services, provided by the NHS and councils to ensure effective diagnosis, treatment and support, for them and their carers."*

Standard 7 was developed partly because:

- The annual direct cost to the NHS of caring for people with AD was estimated at over £1 billion in 1993. The costs to other agencies and the costs of informal carers mean that the total cost may be £6 billion a year.
- There is considerable regional variation in the availability of services.
- Mental health problems in older people often remain undetected.

Two other standards in the NSF for Older People are also relevant to AD:

- Standard 2: *"NHS and social care services treat older people as individuals and enable them to make choices about their own care..."* This means that their dignity and privacy should be respected (including personal hygiene needs), and their need to be involved in decisions about their care should be recognised.
- Standard 8: *"The health and well-being of older people is promoted through a co-ordinated programme of action led by the NHS with support from councils."* This includes educational activities, and creative and social pursuits (see Table A1). The stated aim is to prevent or delay the onset of, or reduce the impact of, ill health and

Reminiscence or art therapy
News-based discussions
Aromatherapy
Games and quizzes
Adult education
Drama

Table A1. Examples of activities that the NSF for Older People says should be offered in residential care, nursing homes, and day care.

disability. This standard also mentions the need for an appropriate – safe, accessible, and stimulating – living environment, with good quality design, lighting, and colour contrast.

The NSF for Older People also makes formal statements on:

- The need for teamwork and good communication between the different healthcare agencies.
- The need for early and accurate diagnosis of dementia, in terms of access to treatment, and enabling older people and their carers to understand and come to terms with the diagnosis and plan for the future.
- The need for access to specialist care, and a full range of support services (with guidance on when to refer).
- The potential of the newer anti-psychotic drugs for people with dementia.

Details of the NICE guidance on the use of AChEIs

The UK government organization, the National Institute for Clinical Excellence, has recommended that the drugs donezepil, rivastigmine and galantamine should be made available to anyone who needs them, on the NHS, if certain conditions are met (Table A2, see also p. 91).

To arrive at its decision, NICE considered both published and unpublished clinical trial evidence, concluding that:

- AChEIs have not shown clinical effectiveness in patients with an MMSE score <10.
- Some patients, who cannot at present be identified before treatment, do not benefit from AChEIs.

The patient has mild or moderate AD with an MMSE score >12
The diagnosis was made in a specialist clinic
The patient is likely to comply with treatment
Treatment follows further specialist assessment of functioning
Treatment is initiated by specialists (GPs can later take over,
under shared care protocols)
Patients are reviewed after 2–4 months, then every 6 months
thereafter
Their MMSE score and functioning is reassessed at each review
Treatment is continued only if there is evidence of benefit at
each review

Table A2. Conditions that should be met before AChEIs are
prescribed for AD on the NHS.

- Although AChEIs significantly improve scores of global
  outcome and cognitive function, their effects on quality
  of life are harder to prove.
- AChEIs may delay institutionalization. NICE assumes
  that a 12 week delay would save the NHS £4–5,000 a
  person. This would affect carers, but it is not known how.
- The cost-effectiveness of the different treatments cannot
  be compared because of methodological differences
  between studies.

NICE suggests that if all suitable patients are given AChEIs,
the total drug bill to the NHS could be up to £42 million (see
Table A3).

Each year, 30,000 patients in the UK are suitable for a trial of
an AChEI
Each patient is prescribed one drug for 6 months at an annual
cost of £800 per patient, so the total cost to the NHS is £12
million a year
Half of the 30,000 show sufficient response to continue
treatment for 3 years (until their condition becomes severe or
they die of something else)
The additional cost of this group is 15,000 × 2.5 (i.e. 3 years
minus the 6 months already on treatment) × £800, which
means a further cost to the NHS of £30 million a year

Table A3. Assumptions and calculations used to determine the
annual cost to the NHS of using AChEIs.

Index

AD – Alzheimer's disease
APP – Amyloid precursor protein
Page numbers followed by 'f' refer to figures;
page numbers followed by 't' refer to tables.
Please note all index entries refer to Alzheimer's disease
unless otherwise noted.

Alzheimer's Disease

Ralph W Richter MD, FACP

Clinical Professor of Neurology and Psychiatry
The University of Oklahoma College of Medicine

Director, Alzheimer's Disease Research Unit
St John Medical Center

President, Clinical Pharmaceutical Trials Inc.
Tulsa, Oklahoma, USA

Brigitte Zoeller Richter dipl. pharm.

Director, PROMEDAS Company
Basel, Switzerland

Director of Publishing, Clinical Pharmaceutical Trials Inc.
Tulsa, Oklahoma, USA

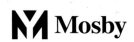

Mosby

MOSBY
An imprint of Elsevier Science Limited.

© 2002 Elsevier Science Limited.

Ⓜ Mosby is a registered trademark of Elsevier Science Limited.

ISBN 0-7234-3263-5

Cataloguing in Publication Data
Catalogue records for this book are available from the US Library of Congress and the British Library.

Note
Medical knowledge is constantly changing. As new information becomes avail-able, changes in treatment, procedures, equipment and the use of drugs become necessary. The editors/authors/contributors and the publishers have taken care to ensure that the information given in this text is accurate and up to date. However, readers are strongly advised to confirm that the information, especially with regard to drug usage, complies with the latest legislation and standards of practice.

Printed by Grafos S.A. Arte sobre papel, Spain.